D0363206

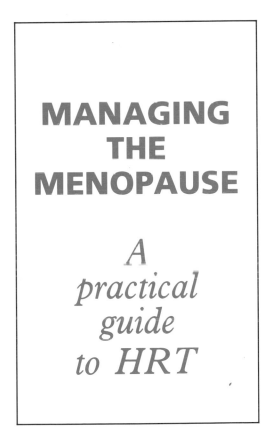

MANAGING THE MENOPAUSE

A practical guide to HRT

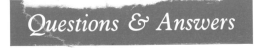

Questions & Answers

The views expressed in this publication are those of the authors and participants and are not necessarily representative of the views of Novo Nordisk Pharmaceuticals Ltd.

Full prescribing information on any product mentioned should be consulted before use.

Further information is available on request from:

Novo Nordisk Pharmaceuticals Ltd
Broadfield Park
Brighton Road
Crawley
West Sussex
RH11 9RT

Novo Nordisk A/S
Novo Alle
DK-2880
Bagsvaerd
Denmark

Tel: 0293 613555

Tel: 010 45 44 44 88 88

ISBN 1-873499-00-0

First published in the United Kingdom by Medical Communications Services, Oxted, RH8 0TF, UK, under an educational grant from Novo Nordisk Pharmaceuticals Ltd.

CONTENTS

Page   Section

CONTENTS

INTRODUCTION

Patient awareness of, and demand for, hormone replacement therapy (HRT) is increasing. Clinicians are therefore under pressure to prescribe treatment more frequently. In view of this it is perhaps surprising that there is so little written which provides a structured approach to treatment and practical prescribing advice.

The idea for this publication was born out of a National Symposium series of some 22 regional meetings entitled "Hormone Replacement Therapy - Time for Reappraisal" which took place between November 1989 and October 1990 throughout Great Britain.

A number of key United Kingdom opinion leaders in the menopause field participated, as speakers, in the meeting series, which was sponsored under an educational grant from Novo Nordisk Pharmaceuticals Ltd, to discuss current issues in the use of HRT.

Prior to each meeting the delegates were invited to submit important topics for discussion; there is little doubt that the 2000 or more replies received represent one of the most comprehensive surveys of current concerns on prescribing HRT in UK general practice. Audience discussions at the meetings demonstrated an overwhelming need for practical advice on a variety of prescribing issues. Answers to the many questions posed were given by the expert opinion present* and a summary of these answers forms the basis of this handbook.

Our aim in this publication has been to provide a practical prescribing guide for doctors. Each of the sections represents an area of controversy, or discussion, about management, which arose during the meeting series. We hope that the format will facilitate the use of this publication as a handbook, and that the references and diagrams included will indicate the published information on which the opinions and advice are based.

Mr N C Siddle

Dr M A Knight

*see overleaf

The Speakers at the National Symposium Series

Mr P Bowen-Simpkins, Consultant Obstetrician and Gynaecologist, Singleton Hospital, Swansea.

Professor D H Barlow, The Nuffield Department of Obstetrics and Gynaecology, John Radcliffe Infirmary, Oxford.

Dr R H Francis, Consultant Physician, The General Hospital, Newcastle upon Tyne.

Dr V A Godfree, Deputy Medical Director, Amarant Trust, Churchill Clinic, London.

Dr D McKay Hart, Consultant Obstetrician and Gynaecologist, Stobhill Hospital, Glasgow.

Mr A D Parsons, Consultant Obstetrician and Gynaecologist, Hospital of St Cross, Rugby.

Professor D W Purdie, Director of Postgraduate Medical Studies, Hull Royal Infirmary, Hull.

Mr N C Siddle, Consultant Obstetrician and Gynaecologist, University College Hospital, London.

Mr J W W Studd, Consultant Obstetrician and Gynaecologist, King's College Hospital, London.

Mr D W Sturdee, Consultant Obstetrician and Gynaecologist, Solihull and East Birmingham Hospital, Birmingham.

Mr M I Whitehead, Consultant Obstetrician and Gynaecologist, King's College Hospital, London.

2 WHY PRESCRIBE HRT?

2.1 What is the pattern of symptoms at the menopause?

Most major complaints during the menopausal period are of subjective symptoms (Figure 1) which peak at around the age of 50 years but begin to occur in women during their 40s.[1] These are the result primarily of changes in circulating levels of oestrogen (Figure 2).[2] It is therefore natural that the frequency and severity of symptoms are subject to individual variation.

Figure 1. Time scale for oestrogen deficiency symptoms. Acute symptoms are followed by symptoms related to the tissue changes which result from prolonged oestrogen deficiency. Osteoporosis and cardiovascular disease become evident 10-15 years after ovarian failure.

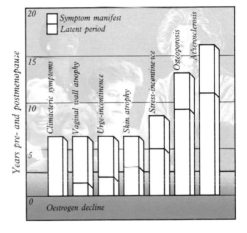

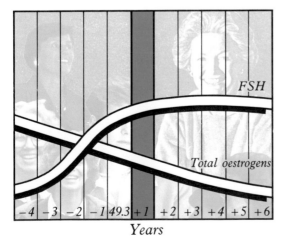

Years

Figure 2. Changes in oestradiol and gonadotrophin levels around the time of the menopause. Follicle stimulating hormone (FSH) and oestrogen levels are related to a time scale where the average age at menopause (49.3 years) is taken as time zero. Oestrogen levels decline from approximately five years before ovarian failure. As the ovarian production of oestrogens declines the pituitary production of FSH rises due to a negative feedback mechanism.

It has been reported that at least 82 per cent of menopausal women experience acute oestrogen deficiency-related symptoms for more than one year[3] and that in 25 per cent of women these symptoms last for more than five years. In addition, 70 per cent of women experience vasomotor symptoms for at least two years and of those who experience severe vasomotor symptoms many have flushes throughout the day.[4] Thus, contrary to popular opinion, these symptoms are neither transient nor occasional. Also, of those women who experience symptoms 51 per cent suffer severely, 33 per cent moderately and 16 per cent mildly (Figure 3).[4]

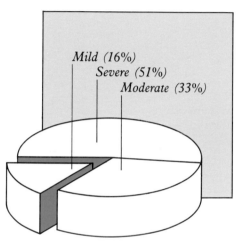

Mild (16%)
Severe (51%)
Moderate (33%)

Figure 3. *The percentage of women who experience severe menopausal symptoms.*[4]

Vasomotor symptoms and sleep disturbance are the most important, and also the most easily recognized, symptoms of oestrogen deficiency because of the profound life disturbance that they cause and because of their acute and severe pattern of onset.

In contrast, other menopausal symptoms arise gradually after a period of oestrogen deficiency and may, at first, be attributed to ageing or to other causes. A good example of this is joint stiffness, which may be confused with primary joint problems and not correctly attributed to the menopause.

The majority of these latter symptoms are caused by tissue changes which result from oestrogen deficiency. These include loss of collagen in skin and ligaments, reduction in blood flow and the slower transmission of nerve impulses. Depending on the part of the body concerned these can produce significant changes in function.

The most marked symptoms caused by tissue changes will occur in the genital tract and bladder with alterations in sexual function and urinary symptoms. Thus, poor arousal and lubrication, loss of sensation and less frequent orgasm often limit sexual enjoyment; urgency, nocturia and reduced resistance to leakage reflect oestrogen deficiency in the bladder and urethra. More general symptoms include loss of muscle strength and muscle mass and, in the central nervous system, a reduction in short-term memory. Irritability, anxious or depressed mood and loss of confidence also occur.

A keen awareness of the broad spectrum of effects associated with oestrogen deficiency is particularly important when treating menopausal women. In this age group symptoms such as tiredness, poor sleep or depressed mood should be recognized as part of the menopausal symptom complex and should not be treated independently. Oestrogen replacement treatment will often produce rapid and complete resolution of a multiplicity of these symptoms (see Section 2.2).

It is particularly important not to misinterpret menopausal symptoms as a manifestation of psychiatric illness or as a part of the ageing process. Where there is doubt a trial of oestrogen treatment is a useful strategy. Generally, three months of treatment with an adequate oestrogen dose will clearly distinguish oestrogen-related symptoms from those due to other causes.

2.2 What is the efficacy of HRT?

HRT is remarkably effective in the treatment of menopausal symptoms. In addition to studies which have shown relief of vasomotor symptoms,[5,6] a large double-blind, placebo-controlled crossover study has demonstrated significant improvement in a variety of psychological and sexual symptoms.[2]

A short-term crossover study of conjugated equine oestrogens with placebo[2] has also demonstrated significant improvements in both physical and psychological symptoms. It is clear from these studies that treatment with oestrogen is substantially better than treatment with placebo.

The range of symptoms for which oestrogen is an effective treatment is extremely broad and includes flushes, depression, insomnia, palpitations, formication, breast pain and loss of ability to concentrate. HRT has proved to be successful in the treatment of these symptoms in 90 per cent of users.[7]

There is also convincing evidence that oestrogen replacement is more effective than placebo in improving the symptoms of voiding difficulties, urinary frequency and urinary urgency that are often experienced by postmenopausal women.[8] Given this, it is perhaps surprising that under 10 per cent of women are currently prescribed any form of hormone replacement.

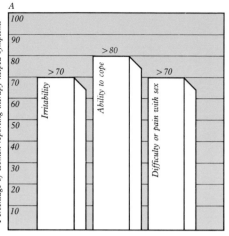

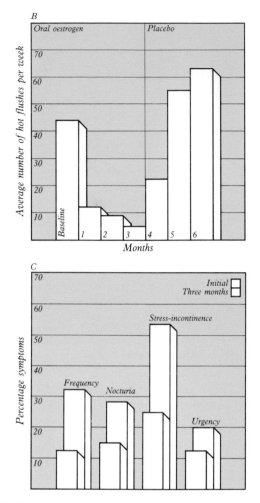

Figure 4. Effectiveness of HRT in relieving symptoms. A. The percentage success in treating irritability, inability to cope and difficulty or pain with sex in a survey of 3117 women on HRT, showing that symptom relief is obtained in over 70 per cent of cases.[7] B. Effect of oestrogen treatment on the number of hot flushes experienced per week (cross-over study).[5] C. Effect of 100 mg oestradiol implant on lower urinary tract symptomatology after three months in 34 women expressed as a percentage of those experiencing symptoms.[8]

Alternative treatments are extremely disappointing. For example, clonidine, which has been recommended for the treatment of hot flushes, fails to achieve effects much greater than those of placebo and, of course, has no effect on any of the other symptoms described.[9]

The use of oestrogen, either alone or in combination with a progestogen, is the most effective treatment for the relief of all menopausal symptoms and all menopausal, i.e. oestrogen-dependent, symptoms will respond to oestrogen treatment provided that an adequate level of replacement is achieved. Where menopausal symptoms do not respond to oestrogen treatment this is usually because of pharmacokinetic problems (see Section 3.4).

The striking effectiveness of HRT is also evident in the treatment and prevention of the long-term sequelae of the menopause — cardiovascular disease and osteoporosis.

There is substantial evidence that oestrogen replacement treatment prevents bone loss[10] and in some cases can increase bone density.[11] Prevention of bone loss with HRT reduces the incidence of osteoporotic fractures[12,13] and potentially lowers the mortality rate from osteoporotic hip fracture[14] (Figure 5). This is an important benefit of treatment since almost one-half of all women who develop osteoporosis sustain some sort of osteoporotic fracture.[15]

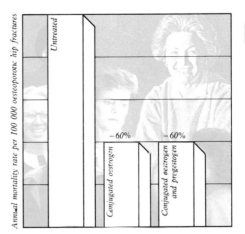

Figure 5. Reduction in mortality with oestrogen treatment. The histograms compare mortality (rate/100 000) in untreated women with that following unopposed or opposed oestrogen treatment (0.625 mg). Both treatments are estimated to reduce mortality by 60 per cent in women aged 65-74.[13]

Oestrogen treatment has a beneficial effect both on cardiovascular mortality (see the review of prospective studies by Vessey and Hunt[16]) and on the severity of coronary occlusion in women with angiographically confirmed ischaemic heart disease. This latter effect is shown in Figure 6 which compares the severity of coronary occlusion stratified according to oestrogen use. There is, therefore, a consensus that oestrogen replacement treatment is protective against ischaemic heart disease leading to at least a 50 per cent reduction in likely mortality.[17-20] A similar protective effect of oestrogen treatment against stroke has been shown in a Californian study.[21]

Thus for both ischaemic heart disease and stroke the protective effect of oestrogen results in a greater than 50 per cent reduction in associated mortality. There is more than one mechanism underlying this effect which will include effects on lipids, blood flow and vasodilatation.[23]

However, the hypothesis raised by Ross et al,[14] and based on epidemiological rather than scientific data, is that combined treatment will have less cardioprotective effect than that seen with unopposed oestrogen treatment.

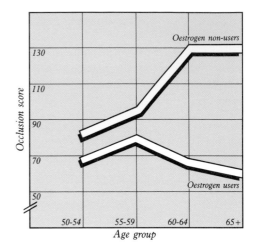

Figure 6. Effects of oestrogen on coronary occlusion. Coronary occlusion score in different age groups of women with angiographically proven ischaemic heart disease showing consistently lower mean scores in those taking oestrogen compared with non-users regardless of age.[22]

Unfortunately this hypothesis is based upon two false assumptions. Firstly, that beneficial lipid effects are the only, or the most significant, mechanism whereby oestrogens exert their cardiac effect and, secondly, that current prescribing practice involves the use of high doses of 19-nortestosterone-derived progestogens (e.g. norethisterone 10 mg) such as reported in the data of Hirvonen et al.[24]

In fact, modern combined regimens have essentially neutral effects on the lipoprotein pattern because they contain only small doses of progestogen (e.g., norethisterone acetate 1 mg)[25] and current opinion suggests that the cardioprotective effect of combined treatment is complex and not simply due to an effect on the lipid profile.[23]

Even when apparently adverse lipid effects are generated on treatment, the overall cardioprotective effect may be beneficial, presumably because of other oestrogen-mediated benefits.[26]

This observation of the effects of oestrogens on cardiovascular and cerebrovascular disease is recent and not yet fully explained. It is undoubtedly a real phenomenon, but it is not clear whether the observed beneficial effects cease immediately upon withdrawal of treatment or whether these protective effects will continue to some extent after treatment has ceased.

2.3 How to assess menopausal symptoms effectively.

For the prescribing doctor the full assessment of those patients who will benefit from treatment with HRT is a key challenge in daily practice. As discussed in Section 2.1 there is a wide range of menopausal symptoms, most of which can be treated effectively (Table 1). It is necessary to determine the range of any one patient's symptoms to decide the most appropriate form of treatment, in terms of both type and duration of use.

Table 1 - MENOPAUSAL SYMPTOMS TREATED EFFECTIVELY WITH HRT

Hot flushes	Mood changes	Genital tract atrophy	Dry thin skin
Night sweats	Anxiety	Dyspareunia	Dry hair
Insomnia	Irritability	Loss of libido	Formication
Palpitations	Poor memory	Increased urinary	Aches and pains
Headaches	Poor concentration	frequency	in joints
Panic attacks	Loss of confidence	Increased urgency	
	Indecisiveness	Nocturia	
	Depression	Dysuria	
	Tiredness/loss of energy		

The provision of a simple questionnaire (see Section 10), which can be completed by the patient, or by the practice nurse on the doctor's behalf, prior to consultation, is a useful approach which will ensure that the patient discloses those symptoms which she is experiencing both comprehensively and concisely.

An accurate assessment of the information obtained will facilitate selection of the correct treatment approach with the minimum time expenditure. The choice of treatment is discussed further in the next chapter.

3 STARTING TREATMENT

3.1 How long to treat: Strategies.

How long to treat

Although no consensus exists on the optimal duration of oestrogen replacement treatment, it is possible to construct a logical framework. Acute menopausal symptoms, particularly vasomotor symptoms, occur for between one and five years in 56 per cent of women (see Section 2.1) and for more than five years in 26 per cent of women (Figure 7).[3]

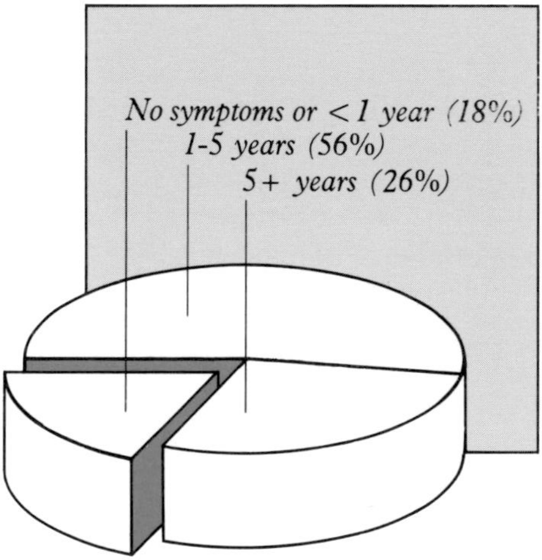

No symptoms or < 1 year (18%)
1-5 years (56%)
5+ years (26%)

Figure 7. *Average duration of menopausal symptoms experienced by those women who suffer.*

Although doubts may exist about long-term prophylactic treatment, for 10 or more years, it is clearly reasonable to treat symptomatic women for as long as it is necessary. In this context it is important to remember that more women than previously recognized experience long-term symptoms and that 10 per cent of these will continue to have vasomotor or urogenital symptoms into their 60s.[27]

All too frequently, when a patient presents with menopausal symptoms, an inappropriately short course of HRT is prescribed (two to three months) and then withdrawn at the patient's request, or the doctor's insistence, because its effectiveness has not been convincingly demonstrated. This is not a reasonable approach. Equally, it is extremely unkind to start a symptomatic woman on treatment, relieve her symptoms for a period of two to three months and then withdraw treatment, provoking an acute recurrence of symptoms.

Thus it is essential that an appropriate management strategy be planned once the menopause has been identified as the cause of the symptoms and the decision to treat has been made. Various strategies are applicable; the initial choice will depend upon whether the patient simply requires symptomatic relief or has been assessed at the outset to require long-term treatment, e.g. for the prevention of osteoporosis.

Strategies

Symptom Relief — Short- and Medium-Term Strategies

1. Treatment for two to three years to provide symptom relief, after which treatment can be gradually withdrawn provided that symptoms do not recur.

2. Treatment for two to three years to provide symptom relief. Where the withdrawal of treatment leads to a recurrence of symptoms, treatment should be continued until it can be withdrawn without effect.

3. Treatment for two to three years to provide symptom relief, after which time the patient does not wish to withdraw from treatment because of improved well-being and/or a wish for preventive treatment because of a family history of, or fears about, osteoporosis or cardiovascular disease. Treatment should then be discussed and continued, if appropriate, for a further three to eight years, when a further review of strategy can be undertaken.

Prophylaxis against Osteoporosis and Cardiovascular Risk —
Long-Term Strategies

4. Decide at the outset to treat long-term (for at least five years and probably ten years) for the prevention of osteoporosis because either this course of action is specifically indicated or has been requested by the patient.

These are the main strategies and it is helpful to note at the outset which of these is proposed.

In certain cases it may be appropriate to begin long-term treatment at the outset (see Section 3.2). It is also quite appropriate to begin with symptomatic treatment and then to make a decision about long-term treatment after the woman has been treated for two to three years.

In the case of most of these strategies, withdrawal from treatment will be necessary at some stage. When this is appropriate, it is best, in consultation with the patient, to effect a planned withdrawal of treatment to minimize any

11

symptom recurrence, particularly in the case of short-term treatment. This is best achieved by reducing the dose of oestrogen gradually over a period of several months. During this time the progestogen dose should be maintained.

When treatment is provided in the form of a combination pack, one of the simplest approaches is to reduce the administration of once-daily oestrogen to alternate-daily administration, for instance by omitting every other tablet, whilst continuing the full progestogen course.

3.2 When is long-term treatment justified?

There are many instances where there is a clear indication that a woman will justifiably benefit from long-term treatment.

The patient in whom symptomatic atrophic genital tract changes have been reversed, or in whom a urinary continence procedure or prolapse repair has been performed successfully, is an obvious candidate for long-term treatment. This will maintain the benefit of treatment or surgery and prevent atrophy or a recurrence of prolapse and incontinence. Similarly the patient who presents with established osteoporosis, a family history of osteoporosis, or coronary heart disease is also a candidate for long-term treatment.

Women with a premature menopause, either idiopathic or surgical, are a particularly important group that must be given long-term treatment. This is because the consequences of both increased cardiovascular risk and loss of bone and collagen occurring early in life are potentially catastrophic. For example, there is a four- to five-fold increase in the risk of myocardial infarction in women with premature ovarian failure[28] in an age group where ischaemic heart disease is rare.

In terms of osteoporosis, premature ovarian failure will advance the age at which this condition occurs and therefore the likelihood of fracture occurrence.[29]

If we assume that susceptible individuals reach their theoretical fracture threshold 10-15 years after ovarian failure it is clear that women who become menopausal before the age of 40 will be at risk of fracture in their 50s. This will have dramatic medical and social consequences.

3.3 What type of HRT regimen is recommended?

Today, for the majority of women with an intact uterus a combined treatment regimen should be prescribed. However, treatment can take the form of oestrogen tablets that contain either natural oestrone, oestradiol or equine oestrogens that are given regularly for three weeks out of every four (cyclic unopposed), or continuously (continuous unopposed) (Figure 8). These were the usual forms of treatment up until the late 1970s.

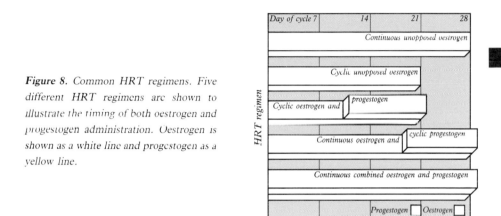

Figure 8. *Common HRT regimens. Five different HRT regimens are shown to illustrate the timing of both oestrogen and progestogen administration. Oestrogen is shown as a white line and progestogen as a yellow line.*

If cyclical oestrogen is given without progestogen addition, up to 25 per cent of women will experience episodes of bleeding,[30,31] although this will not necessarily follow any regular pattern and may occur in the treatment-free week or at other times. With this particular regimen the presence or absence of bleeding gives no indication of the normality of the endometrium, or of the presence of any premalignant or malignant changes.[30,32,33]

Seven to 15 per cent of women taking oral oestrogen alone will develop endometrial hyperplasia[32-34] which is dose- and duration-dependent. The proportion of those hyperplasias which will progress to malignancy depends on the degree of cellular atypia present at the time of sampling.[35] However, there is no doubt that this type of treatment is associated with a definite increase in the incidence of endometrial cancer. A review of the available literature suggests that the incidence is between two and nine times greater than that in the untreated population.[36]

It is now accepted that small doses of progestogen should be given with oestrogen treatment for a defined period each month. Such combination treatment (cyclic opposed) has been shown to reduce the risk of endometrial cancer to below that seen in the untreated population.[37,38]

The use of oestrogen-only treatment is now usually reserved for those women who have had a hysterectomy, or for the very small number of women who, for various reasons, cannot tolerate progestogens. In this latter group specialist surveillance is required, with endometrial biopsy at least every twelve months or whenever bleeding occurs.

Unfortunately, the disadvantage of any cyclic opposed regimen is that most patients will experience the re-establishment of withdrawal bleeding. Whilst this side effect does appear to be well-tolerated by most women, those older women requesting long-term treatment for protection against postmenopausal bone loss are less likely to tolerate the re-establishment of bleeding.

To overcome this, attempts have been made to develop a treatment which produces an atrophic endometrium and thus amenorrhoea.

This has taken the form of a continuous combined oestrogen and progestogen regimen in which progestogen is taken continuously, every day, in combination with the oestrogen (continuous combined). The most successful regimen designed so far is a combination of oestradiol (2 mg) with norethisterone acetate (1 mg).[39]

Whilst the mechanism by which continuous progestogen administration renders the endometrium atrophic has not been fully elucidated, the picture seen is similar to that in premenopausal women receiving continuous progestogens or a highly progestogenic combination, e.g. the progestogen-only pill, depot progestogen injection or the combined oral contraceptive pill.[40]

Early reports have been encouraging, with more than 96 per cent of patients developing an atrophic endometrium. However, 40 per cent of patients experienced light but irregular bleeding during the first treatment month, with approximately 10 per cent still bleeding during the fourth month.[41,42]

It may therefore be that some treatment modifications are needed before this regimen can be used effectively in general practice. Experience with other regimens has been reviewed by Whitehead et al.[39]

3.4 What type of oestrogen should be prescribed?

Oestrogens are usually described as either natural or artificial. Of those oestrogens that are found in commonly prescribed HRT preparations, 17β-oestradiol, oestriol, oestrone and the conjugated equine oestrogens equilin and 17α-dihydroequilenin are of 'natural' origin (Table 2).

17β-oestradiol, oestriol and oestrone are the naturally occurring human oestrogens. By contrast, conjugated equine oestrogens are extracted from the urine of pregnant mares and contain a mixture of oestrone, equilin, 17α-dihydroequilenin and their respective sulphates and glucuronides.[43]

Table 2 - TYPES OF OESTROGEN

NATURAL	ARTIFICIAL
17β-oestradiol	Ethinyl oestradiol
Oestradiol valerate	Mestranol
Oestrone piperazine sulphate	Diethylstilboestrol
Conjugated equine oestrogens	Dienoestrol
(equilin + 17α-dihydroequilenin)	
Oestriol	

To date no-one has produced any comparative data to show that one form of natural oestrogen is better than any another, either in terms of relief of symptoms, side-effect profile or any adverse long-term consequences.

17β-oestradiol is the principal circulating oestrogen. It is produced from the premenopausal ovary by the conversion of testosterone in granulosa cells, whilst oestrone, the second major naturally-occurring oestrogen, is derived both from the metabolism of 17β-oestradiol and the aromatization of androstenedione in adipose tissue.

Because of very rapid glucuronidation in the circulation, oestriol administration produces little systemic oestrogen effect. The use of oestriol is therefore restricted mainly to vaginal preparations designed to achieve vaginal oestrogenization without any generalized systemic effect.

In postmenopausal women the only natural circulating oestrogen arises from the aromatization of androstenedione and testosterone in adipose tissue, skin

15

and liver. Androstenedione and testosterone continue to be produced by the ovarian stroma and adrenal cortex even when the ovary has ceased to secrete oestrogen.

With the exception of those preparations containing conjugated equine oestrogens most oral preparations of HRT now contain 17β-oestradiol, oestrone, or esters of these which are metabolized to natural oestrogen within the body (Figure 9). Although the natural oestrogens are not as potent as their artificial alternatives, e.g. stilboestrol, ethinyl oestradiol and mestranol, which are the most commonly used agents in oral contraceptives, the natural oestrogens are effective and produce fewer side effects.[44]

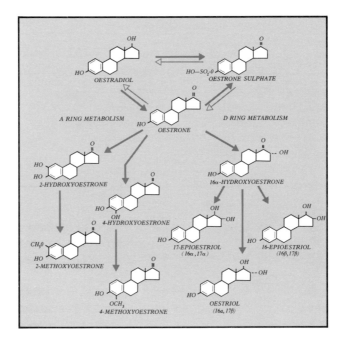

Figure 9. The routes of metabolism of the natural oestrogens and their metabolites.

The artificial oestrogens, shown in Table 2, have a profound effect on the liver. This is partly because the potency of the contraceptive doses used is significantly higher than that of natural oestrogens in HRT, but also because ethinyl oestradiol is not metabolized in the liver. Hence it remains bound to hepatocyte oestrogen receptors for a longer period of time, thus exerting more prolonged effects (Figure 10).[45]

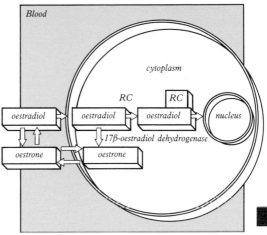

Figure 10. *The dynamics of oestrogen turnover in cells of target tissues. Oestradiol, the principal intracellular form of oestrogen, which diffuses into the cell, is bound to the oestrogen receptor (RC) and transported into the nucleus. The effect of oestradiol is limited by the action of 17β-oestradiol dehydrogenase which converts oestradiol to oestrone. Oestrone has less affinity for the oestrogen receptor. Thus it is retained in the nucleus for a relatively short time and produces less oestrogenic stimulus.*

The pronounced deleterious effects of artificial oestrogens, upon both coagulation factors and carbohydrate tolerance, have been reviewed recently by Upton.[46] Because of these effects, artificial oestrogen should not be prescribed as replacement treatment.

Conjugated equine oestrogens differ from oestradiol and oestrone in some of their actions. This is seen predominantly as a greater potency in hepatic effect,[44] perhaps due to the absence of intracellular enzymatic mechanisms for the metabolism of equine oestrogens such as equilin. This leads to longer retention of oestrogen within the target cells where it is bound to the oestrogen receptor, and thus to a prolonged clinical effect. This occurs to an even greater extent with the artificial oestrogens. However, the clinical significance of this is unclear.

In everyday practice, there is little difference in clinical effect between the natural oestrogens. 17β-oestradiol, the conjugated equine oestrogens and oestrone sulphate appear to be equally effective.[44]

3.5 How should the appropriate dose and route of administration of oestrogen be decided?

During normal ovulatory cycles, ovarian production of 17β-oestradiol ranges from 60-600 μg/day (Figure 11), and results in circulating levels of serum oestradiol from 180-1350 pmol/l. After menopause, the ovarian production rate of 17β-oestradiol is less than 20 μg/day and circulating levels in the serum are less than 150 pmol/l.

17

The specific aim of HRT is therefore to produce serum oestradiol levels that approach premenopausal levels in women for whom ovulatory function has either declined or ceased. This should effectively relieve symptoms and also protect against osteoporosis.[15] Care should be taken to ensure that women are not treated with doses that simply relieve most of these symptoms but do not protect the skeleton (see Section 8.3).

Figure 11. *Comparison of the mean oestradiol concentration in plasma during the menstrual cycle with mean concentrations obtained after administration of exogenous oestradiol by various routes. Oestradiol levels peak mid-cycle prior to ovulation. Horizontal lines represent mean plasma levels obtained following a 50 mg oestradiol implant, a 100 μg transdermal patch, a 50 μg transdermal patch and oral doses of 1 mg and 2 mg oestradiol (data from Campbell and Whitehead[47]).*

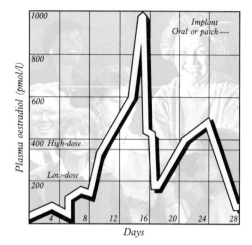

Oestrogens can be administered orally, transdermally or vaginally. In general, vaginal routes are not widely used clinically, except for treatments that are designed to produce a purely local effect.

17β-oestradiol or oestradiol valerate is usually given orally in doses of 1-4 mg daily. An approximate clinical equivalence is 0.625-1.25 mg of oral conjugated equine oestrogens, 1.5-3.0 mg of oestrone sulphate or 0.05-0.1 mg of 17β-oestradiol transdermally[48] (Figure 12).

When compared with equine oestrogen, the dose of oral 17β-oestradiol that is required to produce an equivalent serum oestradiol level is significantly higher than that of the conjugated equine alternatives. This is because unconjugated oestradiol is rapidly metabolized and inactivated in the liver.

By contrast, transdermal absorption produces appropriate and clinically effective serum levels of 17β-oestradiol at much lower doses (0.05 mg or 0.1 mg) than with oral administration. This is because transdermal oestradiol avoids the first pass effect through the liver (see Figure 13). Approximately forty times as much oestradiol must be given orally as transdermally,[48] quantifying the effects of the enterohepatic recirculation and first pass mechanism (Figure 13).

Figure 12. Comparison of pre- and postmenopausal mean oestradiol plasma levels with those produced by different treatment modalities. The histograms show plasma oestradiol in the menstruating premenopausal woman and the fall that occurs postmenopausally. These treatment routes and doses are compared with the endogenous oestradiol levels, oral 1 and 2 mg daily, transdermal 100 μg daily and implant 25 mg six-monthly.[49]

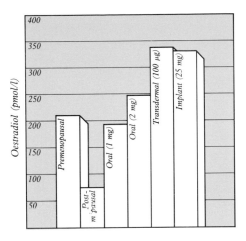

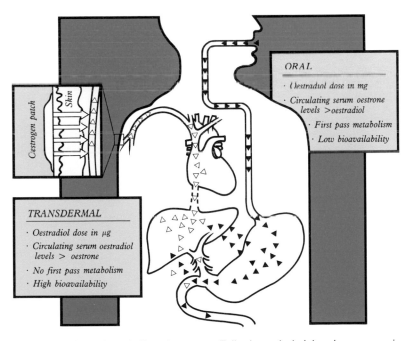

Figure 13. Absorption and metabolism of oestrogen. Following oral administration oestrogen is absorbed into the portal system and passes through the liver before entering the circulation. Following transdermal administration oestrogen passes directly into blood vessels in subcutaneous tissue and is distributed in the body before being influenced by hepatic metabolism.

Finally, in subcutaneous form, pellets of 17β-oestradiol in doses from 25-100 mg can be used. With 25 mg pellets plasma levels between 190 and 782 pmol/l are seen two weeks after implantation and levels of 227-253 pmol/l are maintained for approximately six months.[50] These plasma levels produce good symptom relief. In those pre- and perimenopausal women particularly, who demonstrate low oestrogen levels using 25 mg implants, higher subcutaneous doses may be used, and will be required to provide symptom relief and to suppress ovarian function.[51]

In general, all routes of administration are effective. Thus cost, simplicity and patient administration are the main considerations when choosing treatment. As oral oestrogen is effective, simple and inexpensive, it should be the first line of approach in most circumstances.

Table 3 shows some of the particular circumstances that will dictate the type of treatment to be prescribed. Such circumstances include previous thromboembolism, where it is imperative to minimize hepatic effects (see Section 6.3), where adequate symptom relief has not been achieved due to low plasma oestradiol levels, or where concomitant antiepileptic treatment enhances hepatic metabolism (see Section 6.4).

Table 3 - WHICH PATIENT - WHICH PREPARATION?

Patient	Oral	Implant	Percutaneous/ transdermal	Vaginal
Climacteric symptoms	★	★	★	
First-line treatment	★		★	
Nausea or vomiting		★	★	
Little effect with oral treatment		★	★	
Atrophic vaginitis				★
Diabetic	★	★	★	★
Epileptic		★	★	★
Previous history of thromboembolism		★	★	★

Modified from Cardozo.[51a]

Transdermal oestrogens are useful for those in whom oral treatment is unacceptable or where difficulties are experienced in achieving therapeutic plasma levels due to enhanced liver metabolism. Transdermal or subcutaneous oestrogen administration is also usually preferred in cases where it is important to minimize the hepatic effects of administration,[52] such as in women with a previous history of thromboembolism.

It is common practice to withdraw women from treatment after five to ten years.[53] This is not essential but there will be many women in their mid 60s who are happy gradually to withdraw from treatment, or who will find that the use of much reduced doses of oestrogen will still maintain benefit.

The advantage of the latter approach is that, if the oestrogen dose is reduced and the progestogen dose is continued, many women will cease to experience withdrawal bleeding. This can be a useful approach because, at this stage, having deferred the onset of oestrogen deficiency-related bone and collagen loss for five to ten years or so, it is less critical to use doses of oestrogen that protect fully against bone loss since the onset of fracture has been significantly delayed.

3

3.6 When should a progestogen be used and which type?

The main reason for the sequential addition of a progestogen is to reduce the consequences of unopposed oestrogen administration, namely irregular bleeding and the risk of endometrial hyperplasia and endometrial cancer (see Sections 3.3 and 3.7).

Table 4 - RELATIVE RISK OF ENDOMETRIAL CANCER AFTER EXPOSURE TO TREATMENT ACCORDING TO DURATION OF TREATMENT

A - Oestrogen alone

Duration of treatment (months)	Number of cases observed	Number of cases expected	Relative risk (95 per cent confidence interval)
⩽6	6	5.5	1.1 (0.5-2.5)
7-36	16	11.3	1.4 (0.8-2.4)
37-72	11	9.3	1.2 (0.6-2.2)
⩾73	15	8.2	1.8 (1.1-3.2)
Total	48	34.3	1.4 (1.1-1.9)

B - Oestrogen with cyclically added progestogen

Duration of treatment (months)	Number of cases observed	Number of cases expected	Relative risk (95 per cent confidence interval)
⩽6	0	1.7	0 (0-12.7)
7-36	5	3.6	1.4 (0.5-3.6)
37-72	2	1.7	1.2 (0.3-5.5)
⩾73	0	0.6	0 (0-456.1)
Total	7	7.6	0.9 (0.4-2.0)

This has been confirmed by a recent Swedish study that compared the relative risk of endometrial cancer in women on cyclic unopposed (Table 4) and cyclic opposed (Table 4) treatment.[54] This has demonstrated that the relative risk of endometrial cancer increases with time if unopposed treatment is used, but decreases with time with cyclic opposed treatment.[54]

It has also been suggested that progestogens may protect against breast cancer[37] but this has not been substantiated by other studies.

Although progestogens can have a bone-sparing effect, the duration of progestogen in cyclic opposed regimens is probably too short for any such effect to be exerted.

In summary, although some authors favour unopposed oestrogens,[55] the arguments for opposed treatment are strong. The 25 per cent reported incidence of hysterectomy in women who received five years of treatment with unopposed oestrogens, rising to 28 per cent at the end of follow-up,[56] the increased incidence of endometrial cancer[38,54,57] (Figure 14) and the continuation of increased endometrial cancer risk for up to 14 years after the cessation of unopposed oestrogen treatment[58] are sufficiently potent reasons to recommend the use of cyclic opposed treatment in all women who retain their uteri.

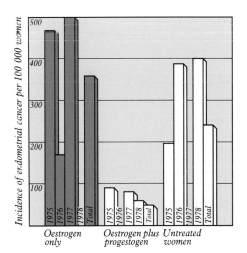

Figure 14. *The effect of opposed or unopposed oestrogen on the incidence of endometrial cancer. Incidence of endometrial cancer/100 000 women is shown for four years observation at Wilford Hall USAF Clinic (1975-1978) for three groups of women: (a) untreated (b) oestrogen only treatment and (c) combined oestrogen and progestogen treatment (7 days).*[37]

The currently recommended regimens use doses of progestogens that are smaller than those used hitherto. Several progestogens are currently available (Table 5).

Table 5 - PROGESTOGENS

19-nortestosterone derivatives	17-hydroxyprogesterone derivatives
Norethisterone acetate*	Medroxyprogesterone
Norethisterone*	Dydrogesterone
Levonorgestrel*	Megestrol acetate
Norgestrel*	Cyproterone acetate
Desogestrel	Medrogestone
Gestodene	
Lynestrenol	
Ethynodiol diacetate	
Norgestimate	
3β-hydroxy desogestrel	
19-norprogesterone	

* Available in opposed HRT preparations in the United Kingdom.

The use of either a 17-hydroxyprogesterone derivative, such as medroxyprogesterone or dydrogesterone, or low doses of a 19-nortestosterone derivative such as norethisterone (1 mg) or levonorgestrel (75 µg), causes minimal metabolic disturbances. These disturbances are unlikely to cause specific problems in their own right or to diminish the cardioprotective benefits produced by unopposed oestrogen treatment (see Section 3.7).

In 80-90 per cent of women the progestogen produces regular monthly bleeding. A variety of side effects, including psychological, physical and metabolic effects, may occur during the progestogen phase or premenstrually and may detract from the benefits of oestrogen treatment.

Approximately 15-20 per cent of women experience minor side effects during the progestogen phase of treatment although less than five per cent are completely intolerant of all types of progestogens. Most women who experience particular problems with one type of progestogen will benefit from a change to a different type.

Progestogen side effects are thought to be dose-related and often a dosage reduction will minimize the intensity and frequency of premenstrual-like symptoms.[59] Regardless of any ill-effects it is essential that the full progestogen course is taken.

3.7 What dose and duration of progestogen is appropriate?

Duration is probably more important than dose when evaluating the addition of progestogen to oestrogen replacement treatment. Early regimens contained seven days of progestogen but it is now known that there is a clear duration effect upon the proliferative status of the endometrium which is independent of dose. In the study of Sturdee et al, 10-13 days of progestogen eliminated endometrial abnormalities completely, whereas a seven day regimen did not.[33] In the case of early combination treatments there was an unacceptable incidence of hyperplasia and, potentially, endometrial cancer. Whitehead et al[30] found a four per cent incidence of endometrial hyperplasia with seven day progestogen regimens and reported an unacceptably high level of endometrial stimulation and poor cycle control. It is important to recognize that endometrial protective effects will vary depending on the oestrogen dose and type, the progestogen type, its dose and duration, and patient compliance.

It appears that cyclic opposed regimens are effective in reducing the risk of endometrial cancer[54,57] and that this risk continues to reduce with time. After six years of treatment the endometrial risk is negligible.[54] Varma[60] found no cases of atypical hyperplasia in women treated with cyclic opposed HRT for a nine-year period, although there was a marked duration effect. Some cases of cystic hyperplasia were reported with a seven day progestogen regimen, but none were observed with the 10 day progestogen regimen.[60]

Thus, it is current practice to use a cyclic opposed regimen with at least 10 days of progestogen. However, care should be taken to allow for the specific combination of oestrogen and progestogen used and, where possible, combinations which have been shown to have proven effects should be selected. This approach has been shown to halve the incidence of endometrial stimulation previously reported with a seven day treatment regimen.[61]

In an attempt to minimize the incidence and severity of side effects which are known to be dose-dependent,[62] dose-ranging studies were undertaken, particularly by Whitehead's group at King's College, London, to establish the minimum dose of progestogen that would provide both endometrial protection and good cycle control.

The first concept tested was to determine whether similar efficacy could be achieved when the progestogen dose was lowered.[63] Subsequently, various doses and different drugs were evaluated (Table 6). This data, based upon endometrial samples taken after six days of progestogen administration, is summarized in the review of Whitehead and Fraser.[31]

Table 6 - ENDOMETRIAL HISTOLOGY IN POSTMENOPAUSAL WOMEN RECEIVING PROGESTOGEN FOR 10-12 DAYS PER MONTH

Progestogen	Atypical hyperplasia (per cent samples)	Secretory endometrium (per cent samples)	Total sample number examined
Norethisterone			
0.35 mg	-	60.0	45
0.7 mg	-	73.1	26
2.5 mg	-	88.2	34
5.0 mg	-	84.6	13
dl-norgestrel			
75 μg	15.8	52.6	19
150 μg	-	73.3	15
500 μg	-	69.6	23
Oral progesterone			
100 mg	33.3	44.4	9
200 mg	-	75.0	16
300 mg	-	85.7	14
Medroxyprogesterone acetate			
2.5 mg	-	40.0	30
5.0 mg	5.9	64.7	17
10.0 mg	-	72.4	29
Dydrogesterone			
5 mg	10.0	54.5	11
10 mg	-	95.2	21
20 mg	-	90.0	10

Oestrogen used = continuous conjugated equine oestrogen 0.625 mg or 1.25 mg daily (Whitehead et al[64]).

A later study with dydrogesterone[65,66] has shown that sampling on day 10 of administration gives a clearer picture and may further validate the use of the low dose regimens suggested by the earlier reviews.

To date, no large scale study has evaluated the risk of endometrial abnormality over finite periods of time with modern combinations. The best available data so far is the study by Paterson et al.[67] Unfortunately, no pretreatment biopsies were performed but the incidence of hyperplasia was extremely low. The only case of hyperplasia seen with 10 days of progestogen treatment reverted to normal without any modification of treatment. Thus, it is clear that the minimum acceptable duration is 10 days and that for each progestogen there is a minimum effective dose which will achieve secretory transformation and prevent hyperplasia. Increasing the dose above this does not significantly increase the effectiveness of treatment.

Thus, for example, with *dl*-norgestrel and dydrogesterone there is little benefit in increasing the progestogen dose above 150 μg and 10 mg respectively. An increase in dose certainly does not increase the percentage of secretory transformation after six days of progestogen (Table 6).

It can be seen from Table 6 that some doses of progestogen will not necessarily induce full secretory transformation. This, in part, reflects the individual variation in bioavailability following oral administration of sex steroids (as discussed in Section 3.8). Padwick *et al*[68] have demonstrated a clinical test for the adequacy of progestogen dose. Those women with poor secretory transformation have poor delay of menstruation and commence the withdrawal bleed early in the progestogen phase of treatment. Conversely, those who have good secretory transformation will not bleed until day 10 or later of the 10-12 day progestogen course (Figure 15).

In clinical practice, therefore, it is important to enquire about the time of onset of withdrawal bleeding. If this consistently occurs before the tenth day of progestogen administration then the dose of progestogen should be increased.

Figure 15. *Secretory transformation of the endometrium on cyclic opposed treatment. Mean day of onset of bleeding after the addition of norethisterone (0.35 mg) or medroxyprogesterone acetate (5 mg) correlated with histology.*[68]

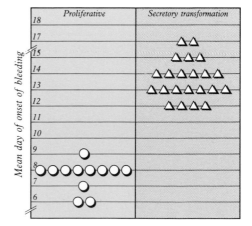

In summary therefore, cyclic opposed regimens should include at least 10 days of progestogen per month and careful attention should be paid to the dose of progestogen administered. Shorter durations of progestogen use will be associated with cases of endometrial abnormality and patients on these regimens should have an endometrial biopsy, perhaps annually. Suitable doses for routine use are shown in Table 7.

Table 7 - MINIMUM ENDOMETRIAL PROTECTIVE DAILY DOSES OF PROGESTOGENS AND DOSAGES USED

Progestogen	Recommended dose	Duration studied (days)	Reference
Dydrogesterone	10 mg	10-12	Lane et al,[69] Varma[60]
Medroxyprogesterone	10 mg	12	Lane et al[70]
Norethisterone acetate	1 mg	10-12	Siddle et al,[63] Varma[60]
Levonorgestrel	75 μg	10-12	Whitehead et al,[64] Varma[60]
Progesterone	200 mg	12	Lane et al[70]

Anecdotal experience from menopause clinics suggests that those women who develop an abnormal endometrium have been poorly compliant with the progestogen phase of treatment. Because of this the use of combination treatment with well-designed packaging, and single daily tablet treatment which does not allow the omission of the progestogen, is particularly advisable in these patients.

3.8 Which route of administration should be chosen?

The choice of treatment is important and the first decision that must be made in this respect is whether to administer oestrogen orally, transdermally by patch or gel, vaginally by cream, pessary or tablet, or subcutaneously. In general, oral administration should be regarded as the first-line option unless a preference is expressed by the patient. It is then important to consider whether to use one of the commercially available combination packs or to combine certain of the separate preparations.

There is no single treatment route that will suit every individual and no one route of treatment is necessarily superior to any other except in exceptional circumstances. For example, epileptic patients who use conjugated oestrogens orally may achieve negligible increases in plasma oestradiol levels[72] due to drug-induced enhancement of liver metabolism, whereas transdermal or subcutaneous administration will produce a therapeutic effect in these patients.

Oral

Oral administration is the most commonly used route of administration due to its simplicity, low cost and familiarity to the patient. However, there is a wide variation in bioavailability because of variable absorption and hepatic metabolism during the first pass enterohepatic recirculation. In addition, it is theoretically possible that the use of high doses of oestrogen given orally could lead to increased hepatic activity, including the production of various lipoproteins, clotting factors and the suppression of circulating natural anticoagulants such as antithrombin III.[73,74] However, usual doses cause little metabolic disturbance (Figure 16) and there is good epidemiological evidence that HRT does not increase the incidence of thromboembolism.[75]

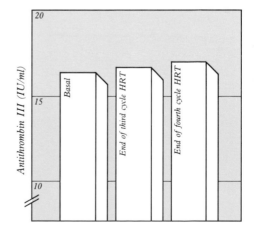

Figure 16. The effect of oral conjugated equine oestrogen (0.625 mg/day) on antithrombin III levels in a selected group of postmenopausal women (n = 12). No significant change was observed.[76]

Implants

Although there have been reports of "tachyphylaxis" to the repeated administration of oestrogen by implant, this is not an exact description of the phenomenon.[77]

With over-frequent repetition of very high oestrogen doses there is a progressive accumulation of oestrogen in body tissues. Thus the body adapts to supraphysiological amounts of oestrogen, and when oestrogen levels fall below this level symptoms of oestrogen deficiency recur. This phenomenon can be avoided by limiting the dose of oestrogen to 25 mg, or perhaps 50 mg, oestradiol and avoiding reimplantation at intervals of less than 20 weeks.

Transdermal

Transdermal administration is used only for the administration of oestrogens at present, but difficulties occur both with skin irritation (19 per cent approximately) and occasionally a significant allergy to the patch adhesive.[78,79]

In addition, hot weather leads to sweating and a reportedly higher percentage of detachment of the patch than normal; in hot climates some racial groups may be prone not only to skin reactions but to significant pigmentation (McCarthy - personal communication).

Whilst both percutaneous and subcutaneous routes have been utilized for the administration of oestrogens, to date the use of these routes for administering progestogens is extremely limited. Whitehead et al[61] have shown that norethisterone can be administered with some success percutaneously, but data on other progestogens are not yet available.

In practice, however, there is no evidence of any major clinical differences between the different routes of administration. There is little doubt that the majority of patients will receive oral HRT at the outset. A number of separate drugs and combinations is available (Table 8).

One of the key issues which should also be considered in the choice of cyclic opposed treatment is patient compliance. The use of combination packs, with well-designed packaging and the inclusion of oestrogen and progestogen in the same tablet, can ensure that the protective effects of the progestogen are never missed.

Table 8 - AVAILABLE OESTROGENS AND COMBINATION PACKS

A - Oestrogen alone

Oestrogen	Dose	Formulation
ORAL		
Conjugated equine oestrogen	0.625-1.25 mg	Combination of oestrone, equilin, equilenin and sulphates, and oestradiol (1-2%)
Oestradiol valerate	1.0-2.0 mg	Ester of 17β-oestradiol
Oestrone piperazine sulphate	1.5 mg	Ester of oestrone
17β-oestradiol, oestrone, etc	Oestriol 0.27 mg Oestradiol 0.6 mg Oestrone 1.4 mg	Combination of natural oestrogens
VAGINAL		
17β-oestradiol	0.025 mg	Tablet
Oestriol	0.01/0.1% 0.5 mg	Cream Pessary
Conjugated equine oestrogens	0.625 mg/g	Cream
Dienoestrol	0.01%	Cream

B - Combined preparations

Oestrogen/ progestogen	Dose	Formulation	Presentation
Oestradiol, oestriol and norethisterone acetate	1.0-4.0 mg 0.5-2.0 mg 1.0 mg	Human oestrogens with 10 days norethisterone acetate	28-day calendar dial pack, one tablet daily
Conjugated equine oestrogens and norgestrel	0.625-1.25 mg 150 μg	Horse-derived oestrogen with 12 days norgestrel	28-day blister pack with two tablets daily during progestogen phase
Oestradiol valerate and *dl*-norgestrel	1.0-2.0 mg 0.25-0.5 mg	Ester of human oestrogen with 10 days *dl*-norgestrel	21-day blister pack, one tablet daily
Mestranol and norethisterone in variable doses	12.5-50.0 μg 0.75-1.5 mg	Synthetic oestrogen with 13 days norethisterone	28-day blister pack, one tablet daily

3

3.9 Initiating treatment.

It is important, at the outset, to identify the motives and expectations of those patients who request HRT, since these are often unrealistic and the patients may have been misinformed about its therapeutic effects or risks. The doctor should establish that patient expectations are reasonable and correct any misunderstandings.

Before starting treatment a full patient history should be taken and a general examination should include height, weight, blood pressure and urinalysis. A breast examination is also essential.

The consultation also represents an ideal opportunity to perform a pelvic examination and cervical smear, if appropriate, at the same time. In the majority of cases both history-taking and the examination can be undertaken by the practice nurse to save valuable consulting time.

It is preferable to start patients on a moderate dose of HRT (e.g. 2 mg oestradiol) to minimize the likelihood of side effects and, for those on cyclic opposed treatment, to discuss and stress the importance of taking the full progestogen course. The nature, timing and purpose of the withdrawal bleed should also be explained, since this is the primary cause of non-compliance in many patients.

The possible occurrence of side effects such as nausea, breast tenderness and leg cramps should be mentioned. Compliance with treatment will be aided if the doctor explains that in those who experience side effects, these will generally subside within the first six to eight weeks of treatment.

Patients should be warned not to expect immediate relief from symptoms. This is particularly vital if the patient's major complaint is of urinary or vaginal symptoms, since the reoestrogenization of tissues generally takes several weeks to occur.

A three month course of treatment should be prescribed. Finally, a follow-up appointment should be arranged at three months to monitor and discuss the suitability of the chosen treatment.

4 MANAGING PATIENTS ON TREATMENT

4.1 How to monitor suitability and type of treatment.

The optimum time to review initial treatment is after an interval of two to three months. There is little point in considering an earlier assessment since although some symptoms, such as hot flushes, begin to improve within the first week of treatment, it may take up to three months before the benefit of treatment is fully established.

There are two reasons for this. The first is that oestrogens induce changes in oestrogen-binding proteins; the second reason is that some of the beneficial effects of HRT result from slowly progressing physical changes such as the revascularization of tissue. For instance, in the genital tract oestrogenization involves the growth of a new, thick, stratified squamous epithelium and the restoration of collagen within the tissues.

As with the prescription of the contraceptive pill it will also take up to three months before the pattern of menstrual bleeding becomes clear, although intermenstrual bleeding will occur quite normally in a proportion of women during the first one or two cycles of HRT.

At the first follow-up visit it is important to assess compliance with treatment as well as its effectiveness and also whether the patient has experienced any adverse effects associated with treatment. In addition, the pattern of bleeding should be reviewed (see Section 4.2) and adjustments made in the dose of oestrogen and/or progestogen to correct any problems which have been identified (Table 9).

Where side effects are observed during cyclic opposed (sequential combined) treatment, the doctor must evaluate the time during the cycle at which these adverse effects occur, since this may provide useful clues about whether they are primarily oestrogenic or progestogenic in origin (see Section 4.3).

Symptoms that occur throughout the cycle may arise from too little or too much oestrogen, whereas effects that are specific to the progestogen phase of treatment are likely to be related to either the type or the dose of progestogen.

Table 9 - FOLLOW-UP INVESTIGATIONS REQUIRED

1. Check symptom control.

2. Enquire about side effects.

3. Enquire about bleeding pattern.

4. Monitor weight and blood pressure six-monthly.

The effectiveness of treatment can be assessed by how well the reported symptoms are relieved. As a general rule, the complete abolition of hot flushes is a good guide that adequate tissue oestrogenization has been achieved (see Section 8.3 for comments on bone protection). Thus, the oestrogen dose should be increased until symptoms are completely abolished. In certain circumstances oestrogen overdose may occur. Symptoms of this include fluid retention, breast tenderness and heavy withdrawal bleeding.

If side effects are experienced only during the progestogen phase of treatment it is worthwhile, firstly, changing the dose, and then changing the drug. The progestogens are a heterogeneous group of drugs that display similar pharmacological actions although they are chemically different. Because of this each may have a different profile of side effects, although the distinctions between the pharmacological effects of the various compounds is poorly understood at the present time.

4.2 Evaluating the withdrawal bleed.

Because this is the major cause of patient withdrawal from sequential combined treatment, and is the side effect which gives the greatest cause for patient concern, considerable emphasis should be placed upon its thorough evaluation at the time of initial review.

It is important that the patient should remember to take the progestogen at a specific time on a regular monthly basis. This can be ensured by clear instruction based on a 28-day cycle (it is helpful to give a written as well as an oral instruction) or by using a calendar pack preparation. This will ensure that the progestogen is taken at the correct time and for the appropriate duration. When using separate drug treatments, such as with an implant or a patch and additional progestogen, the progestogen should be started on the first day of the calendar month since this is easily memorable.

The normal pattern of bleeding in patients on sequential combined treatment is a two to four day light bleed occurring at the end of, or after, the progestogen phase of treatment. Variations from this pattern are important since they may indicate pathology, inadequate oestrogen or progestogen dose or poor compliance. Inevitably, bleeding problems left untreated will lead to poor compliance.

If the history indicates abnormal (heavy or intermenstrual) bleeding it is important to establish first whether the patient is taking her treatment correctly. Where combination packs are used compliance is usually good but difficulties occasionally occur when the treatment is given as two separate tablets.

In general, neither the type of oestrogen nor the type of progestogen will intrinsically lead to abnormal bleeding. If bleeding occurs during the combined phase of sequential treatment, such that the withdrawal bleed occurs early and with no bleeding at any other time, it is probable that the dose of progestogen is inadequate (Figure 17). In such cases the progestogen dose should be increased. If there is any sign that the oestrogen dose is inadequate, such as the continuation of symptoms, then it is appropriate to increase the dose of oestrogen at the same time. Oestrogen plays an important role in priming the endometrium and allows the progestogens to exert their effects. In the case of patients with a very thin atrophic endometrium, too low a dose of oestrogen and the addition of a progestogen may render the endometrium unstable and abnormal bleeding may occur.

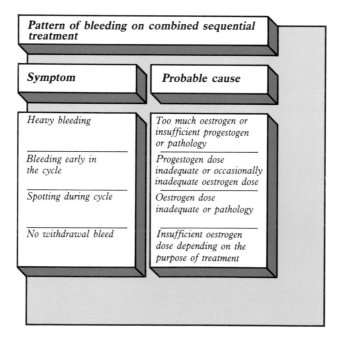

Figure 17. *Probable causes of abnormal bleeding on combined sequential treatment.*

Once it has been established that the patient has been taking her treatment properly and has not omitted the progestogen phase, and dosage adjustments have failed to alter the pattern or extent of bleeding, then pelvic pathology must be excluded (Figure 18). However it is unnecessary to withdraw the patient from treatment until accurate diagnosis has confirmed that this is a necessary course of action.

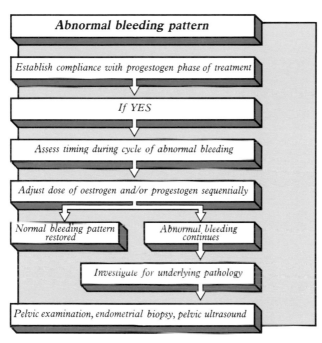

Figure 18. *Investigation and management of abnormal bleeding.*

Pelvic examination, endometrial biopsy and pelvic ultrasound are required to exclude endometrial cancer, endometrial hyperplasia and uterine pathology, such as fibroids or pre-existing ovarian pathology, in particular ovarian cancer.

Bleeding which occurs during the oestrogen-only phase of treatment is much more likely to be associated with pathology than that occurring during the progestogenic phase and should always be investigated. However, where occasional episodes of spotting are reported during the first three months of treatment this should be kept under careful observation and investigated only if the spotting persists.

If withdrawal bleeding is absent and pregnancy has been excluded this is not a cause for alarm, but simply indicates that the oestrogen dose prescribed is low and there is very little endometrial proliferation. In such circumstances it is important, before increasing the oestrogen dose, to review the purpose of treatment. If the main reason for treatment is symptom relief and this is adequate there is no need to increase the oestrogen dose. On the other hand, if treatment has been prescribed to prevent osteoporosis or to oestrogenize the genital tract, then it may be necessary to increase the oestrogen dose to ensure appropriate tissue oestrogenization or to provide skeletal protection.

Delaying the withdrawal bleed
In certain circumstances it may be desirable to delay the normal withdrawal bleed, e.g. when this coincides with a special occasion or holiday. This can be achieved safely by delaying the progestogen course and immediately beginning the next oestrogen phase of treatment. This will delay the withdrawal bleed by one to two weeks. However, this practice should not be adopted by any individual on a frequent or regular basis since prolonged oestrogen-only treatment may lead to abnormal bleeding or endometrial stimulation.

4

4.3 How should side effects be managed?

Side effects experienced by women on a combined HRT regimen are attributable either to too much, or too little, oestrogen or progestogen. The timing of the symptoms, i.e. whether they occur throughout the cycle or only during the progestogen phase, will give an indication of which component is responsible. In each case the doctor must be prepared to be flexible over the adjustment which will be necessary to treatment.

When combined packs are used there is limited flexibility of dose. Certain combination packs exist with different strengths of oestrogen but the progestogen dose is constant. Thus the patient may have to switch to a separate oestrogen and a separate progestogen in order to modify the treatment appropriately. When modifications are made to the regimen it is important to change only one component at any one time, and to evaluate the response before making further changes to treatment.

Too little or too much oestrogen
In general, hot flushes provide the best guide to the adequacy of oestrogenization. Any woman who continues to have hot flushes on treatment can be regarded as essentially undertreated and any other associated symptoms are likely to be due to oestrogen deficiency. However, it is always reasonable to consider a small increase in the dose of oestrogen on a trial basis if there is any doubt about the appropriate course of action. Headaches, formication, lethargy, poor sleep and poor libido will all be improved by increasing the oestrogen dose.

In certain women symptoms of oestrogen overdose may occur. These include heavy bleeding, fluid retention, increased appetite and nausea. This latter symptom may occur in particular with oral administration of oestrogens. In most cases this will resolve naturally during the first few weeks of treatment, but should nausea persist it is best treated by changing the route of administration to a transdermal patch or a subcutaneous implant.

Premenstrual symptoms

There is a cluster of symptoms which effectively mimics the premenstrual syndrome (Table 10).[80]

Table 10 - PREMENSTRUAL-LIKE SYMPTOMS

- Breast pain.
- Fluid retention.
- Bloating.
- Increased appetite.

- Irritability.
- Aggression.
- Anxiety.
- Depression.

Premenstrual-like symptoms are associated exclusively with the progestogen phase of treatment and occur in approximately 10 per cent of women.[61] For the majority of women these symptoms can be minimized by altering the dose of progestogen to the lowest clinically-effective dose as some symptoms are dose-dependent,[59] or, in some instances, by changing the type of progestogen. There are no clear guidelines about which progestogen will be more appropriate in any particular circumstance. In addition, individuals may respond idiosyncratically to different progestogens and an individual woman may prefer one particular drug. Thus it is often appropriate to try a different progestogen.

Nortestosterone-derived or 17-hydroxyprogesterone-derived progestogens
Nortestosterone derivatives, such as norethisterone and norgestrel, or the norethisterone pro-drugs lynestrenol and ethynodiol diacetate, have a mild androgenic, as well as a progestogenic, action. This may lead to side effects such as greasy skin and acne.[39] Although cross-sectional data (Siddle, Hunter and Whitehead - unpublished data) have implied that there are other variations between 19-nortestosterone and 17-hydroxyprogesterone derivatives this has not yet been established by well-controlled studies because of methodological problems.[59] However, irritability may be more common with norgestrel, whereas pelvic heaviness and leg cramps are more common with norethisterone.[59] When a change of progestogen is considered it may be most

appropriate to switch from a 19-nortestosterone to a 17-hydroxyprogesterone progestogen, or vice versa, in order to achieve the maximum chemical difference between any two regimens.

Where fluid retention and bloatedness are present a change of diet (to a low fat, high fibre diet) may be helpful. Vitamin B_6 (50-100 mg/day), which has a mild diuretic effect, is also reportedly of benefit.

If premenstrual-like symptoms continue to be unacceptable then the only recourse is to refer the patient to a specialist clinic where oestrogen-only treatment can be given and monitored appropriately.

Weight gain

Although oestrogen treatment is associated with deposition of fat it does not cause true weight gain in the doses used for replacement therapy.[81] Weight gain is more probably due to fluid retention, improved appetite and well-being and, if persistent, should be controlled with diet.

Heavy bleeding

This may be relieved by decreasing the oestrogen dose and/or increasing the progestogen dose. If symptoms are not satisfactorily relieved by this course of action then the patient should be referred for investigation to determine any underlying pathology (Figure 18). Treatment should be continued until a diagnosis has been confirmed.

Migraine

Migraine may be due to relative oestrogen deficiency or, alternatively, to the effects of progestogens. Recent work (Brass and Sarrell - personal communication) has confirmed this by demonstrating that oestrogens are associated with cerebrovascular vasodilatation and that progestogen addition may lead to vasoconstriction. There is, therefore, a natural balance between the oestrogenic and progestogenic effects that needs to be considered in this clinical context. The administration of progestogens alone may have a vasodilatory effect but this is less than that achieved with oestrogens.

If migraine is linked to the progestogen phase of treatment further enquiry will usually uncover a history of cycle-linked migraine. In such cases an increase in oestrogen dose, reduction of the progestogen dose or the use of an alternative progestogen may be necessary to modify this symptom.

When symptoms persist during the progestogenic phase of treatment only, despite modifications to treatment, then oestrogen-only treatment should be considered and the patient referred to a specialist clinic for surveillance.

Hypertension

In general, blood pressure is either unaffected by the administration of HRT or will decrease.[82] HRT may produce hypertension in a small proportion of women; this is probably the result of either an oestrogenic effect which causes an elevation of renin levels in up to eight per cent of women,[83] or a progestogenic effect that causes an increase in renin, angiotensin II or aldosterone.[83]

These problems are largely theoretical since neither long-term oestrogens, combined oral contraceptive pills nor progestogen-only contraceptive pills with ≤0.35 mg norethisterone[83] are associated with hypertension.

In practice, therefore, hypertension is not a contra-indication to treatment. However, underlying hypertension should be controlled prior to the administration of HRT, because of the reduction in cardiovascular morbidity associated with treatment (Figure 19),[84] and blood pressure control should be checked, as is the usual practice, at regular intervals.

4

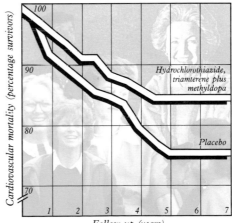

Figure 19. *Effect of active treatment for hypertension on cardiovascular morbidity and mortality. Results are expressed as cumulative per cent survivors without events calculated for the patients on randomized treatment by life-table method.[85]*

4.4. What should be done if patients are unable to tolerate progestogens?

In certain circumstances, such as in those patients who experience migraine during the progestogen phase of combined sequential treatment or unacceptable premenstrual-like symptoms, oestrogen-only treatment should be considered. Fortunately, this occurs in only two to three per cent of patients. However, it is particularly important to identify these patients. They frequently fail to comply with combined sequential treatment once they have indentified that the progestogen phase of treatment is the cause of the unpleasant symptoms they are experiencing and are therefore 'at risk' of developing endometrial abnormality.

Because of the risks associated with endometrial stimulation[58] these women should be referred to specialist clinics for unopposed oestrogen treatment, since an annual endometrial biopsy will be required.

Depending on the dose and duration of the unopposed cyclical oestrogen prescribed the incidence of cystic hyperplasia has been reported to be between seven and 20 per cent [33,86] and, despite regular scheduled withdrawal bleeding, or even in the absence of uterine bleeding, there can be no guarantee that underlying endometrial pathology is not present.

In addition, long-term endometrial surveillance must be continued for a considerable period once treatment has ceased.[58,87]

4.5 What screening is required during treatment?

For the majority of women who have no contra-indications to treatment little screening is required.

There is no evidence that oestrogens significantly increase weight[81] or blood pressure (Figure 20).[82] However, individual women may react idiosyncratically and thus weight and blood pressure should be checked every six months; breast examination should be repeated at 12-monthly intervals (Figure 21). Pelvic examination should be performed at the time of routine cervical cytology, i.e. three-yearly in the UK.

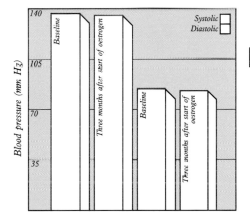

Figure 20. The effect of oral oestrogen on blood pressure in menopausal women. Systolic and diastolic blood pressure (mm Hg) before treatment and after three months of treatment with oral conjugated equine oestrogens. There is no significant change.[82]

Given the high prevalence of breast cancer, women in their 50s should have access to some form of breast screening. This will vary from country to country, e.g. in the UK the government is supporting a policy of three-yearly mammography.

Menopausal women receiving HRT visit their doctor at least annually and this is an ideal time to institute screening. Annual breast examination will identify a small percentage of lesions and two- to three-yearly mammography will identify more. The choice of interval for screening is made on the basis of cost-effectiveness. The number of interval cases will rise as the length of the interval is increased and cost will increase with the frequency of screening. A two-year interval is probably the best compromise when combined with an annual breast examination. Three-yearly intervals, as suggested by Forrest[88] are economic but can increase the number of interval cases. Those women with previous breast abnormalities or dysplasia may require annual mammography.

At present, experience in the UK shows that breast screening is effective in finding breast pathology but that it may be some years before this is translated into evidence of saved lives.[89] This is partly due to the inadequacy of current treatment and partly due to the need for long-term follow-up.

Screening summary

Before treatment	Six-monthly	12-monthly	Three-yearly
Cervical smear	Check weight	Breast examination	Mammography*
Pelvic examination	Check blood pressure	Pelvic examination if cervical cytology required	Pelvic examination
Check blood pressure			
Check weight			
Breast examination			
Mammogram if available			
Bone densitometry if available			

*Unless previous pathology when 12-monthly mammography is advised.

Figure 21. Summary of screening procedures recommended during treatment.

The frequency of screening for cervical cytology is not affected by the use of hormone replacement treatment.

With sequential oestrogen/progestogen regimens endometrial biopsy is not required in the presence of regular withdrawal bleeding or in the absence of uterine bleeding. However, data on the need for biopsy with continuous combined regimens is too sparse for recommendations to be made at present.

PATIENT TYPES

5.1 Perimenopausal women - when should treatment start?

Many women experience vasomotor symptoms when still menstruating, i.e. some years before the menopause. Two studies, in particular, have looked at the prevalence of oestrogen deficiency symptoms prior to ovarian failure. Upton[46] reported that 38 per cent of women aged 40-45 experienced flushes at some time during their menstrual cycle, while Bungay et al,[1] comparing the number of symptoms in men and women around the age of 50, clearly showed that women experience increasing frequency and duration of symptoms as the menopause approaches rather than an acute onset (Figure 22).[1]

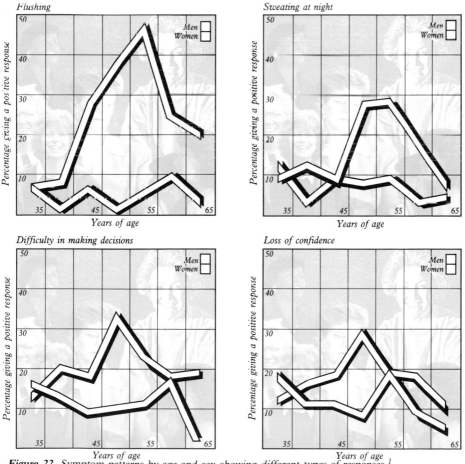

Figure 22. Symptom patterns by age and sex showing different types of responses.[1]

The reason for these symptoms is declining ovarian follicular activity,[90] fluctuations in plasma oestrogen levels, a lower overall level of ovarian secretion and increasing FSH levels.

Once the first rise in FSH levels has been observed the timing to complete ovarian failure is subject to individual variation (Figure 23).[90]

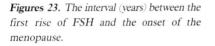

Figures 23. *The interval (years) between the first rise of FSH and the onset of the menopause.*

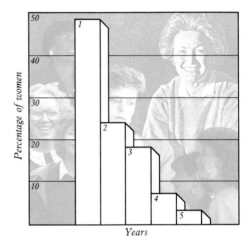

HRT should be given as soon as menopausal symptoms become prevalent. It is best to synchronize combined sequential treatment with the menstrual cycle to ensure that there is adequate oestrogen and progestogen cover through the cycle.[91]

Inevitably, because of the naturally changing hormonal status and the fluctuations which occur in endogenous hormone levels, the degree of symptom relief experienced may vary from month to month. Thus, patients should be counselled that they may experience some irregular bleeding and oestrogenic side effects when these fluctuations occur.

However, this should not be a cause for concern since better hormonal balance, and thus relief of symptoms, will be achieved by treatment in most patients.

A three to six month trial should suffice to demonstrate whether treatment is beneficial to the patient. Treatment can be continued for probably one to two years in the first instance.

5.2 How should premature ovarian failure be treated?

It is particularly important to seek out and treat this group of patients since these women will spend, on average, 20-30 years longer in a postmenopausal state than their healthy counterparts and thus benefit profoundly from treatment. In addition to those women who have had a surgical or idiopathic early menopause there are an increasing number who will have premature ovarian failure as the result of radiotherapy/chemotherapy regimens (Figure 24).

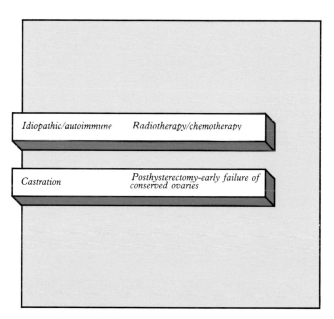

Figure 24. Causes of premature ovarian failure.

These women will often experience severe menopausal symptoms in early life. In the long-term they will also have a dramatically increased risk of coronary heart disease.[92,93] Indeed, some studies have suggested that women with premature menopause or oophorectomy are at a seven-fold greater risk of cardiovascular disease than those with intact ovaries[94] and are also at an increased risk of myocardial infarction.[28]

Significant concerns have also been raised about increased osteoporosis risk in these women since it is clear that it is the time elapsed since menopause, rather than chronological age, which determines skeletal composition (Figure 25). Comparison of bone density in two groups of women, those 20 years past natural menopause (age approximately 70 years) and those 20 years past surgical menopause (age approximately 50 years), reveals no significant difference in loss of bone density.[29]

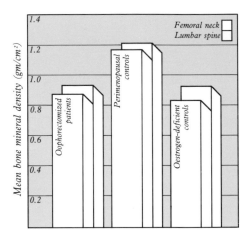

Figure 25. Comparison of the bone density in femoral neck and lumbar spine in three groups of women. Oophorectomized women with mean age of 54 years compared with either age-matched perimenopausal controls (mean age 52) or duration of oestrogen-deficiency-matched controls after natural menopause (mean age 74).[29]

In addition, it is apparent that the rate of trabecular bone loss in women after surgical menopause is 10 per cent, or almost double the rate seen in normal menopausal women.[95]

One important group of patients which should not be overlooked for treatment, and should receive careful attention, are hysterectomized women with intact ovaries. There is now strong evidence to suggest that in up to 24 per cent of these women ovarian failure occurs within two years of surgery and, in most, at least five years before the normal menopausal age due to disruption of ovarian blood supply (Figure 26).[96]

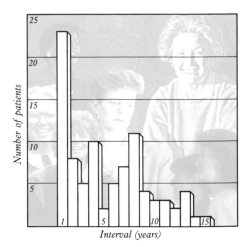

Figure 26. Frequency distribution of interval between hysterectomy with ovarian conservation and clinical or biochemical evidence of ovarian failure in 90 women (<45 years of age at operation). Frequency is skewed to the left, with a significant number of women experiencing ovarian failure surprisingly early after surgery.[96]

Those women who have premature ovarian failure following hysterectomy or oophorectomy can be treated with unopposed oestrogen.

5.3 How should the older postmenopausal woman be treated?

Increasingly there is demand for HRT from older postmenopausal women. If there is evidence of continuing symptoms (e.g. marked tissue changes, such as vaginal atrophy, prolapse or urinary symptoms) HRT should be prescribed for such patients since both genitourinary and bladder symptoms can be reversed.[8]

One of the main drawbacks to treatment in this group is the unacceptability of withdrawal bleeding once the patient has experienced a significant period of amenorrhoea. This can often be dealt with successfully by careful counselling to outline the therapeutic benefits and to encourage motivation and compliance. In addition, many patients who commence treatment in their 60s may not experience withdrawal bleeding (see Section 4.2).

Where withdrawal bleeding does occur and is unacceptable progestogen-only treatment should be considered. For example, norethisterone, 5 mg daily, has been shown to preserve bone[97] and to be more effective than placebo, relieving hot flushes in 70 per cent of women (Figure 27).[98] When using progestogen alone, either because of a wish to avoid withdrawal bleeding or because of concurrent breast cancer, local vaginal application of oestriol[99] or oestradiol (0.025 mg) (data on file) can be used without any systemic effect.

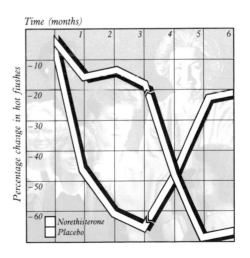

Figure 27. *Norethisterone (5 mg) effectively relieves flushing. This has been demonstrated in a double-blind crossover study.*[98]

Local oestrogen application will help vaginal symptoms. Endometrial proliferation does not occur when oestriol is used orally as a tablet, or vaginally as a cream or pessary, or when oestradiol is used as a vaginal tablet. These treatments are therefore suitable either for use alone for vaginal or bladder symptoms or in addition to progestogen treatment when this is used to preserve bone. It is important to note that local application of conjugated equine oestrogens and orthodienoestrol will cause significant elevation of plasma levels and may cause systemic effects and endometrial proliferation. The use of additional progestogens should be considered with these latter preparations.

In the case of asymptomatic patients with established osteoporosis only little can be done to reverse this process effectively.[100] However, there is convincing evidence that oestrogen treatment, because of its antiresorptive properties, will stabilize bone density in the lumbar spine and femoral shaft.[101] Nevertheless, once oestrogen treatment is discontinued bone resorption continues.[10] Oestrogen treatment should be continued long-term in these patients.

Whilst oestrogen is the preferred treatment in such patients alternative antiresorptive therapies, such as calcitonin[102] or sodium etidronate[20,103,104] have been shown experimentally to be of use in those who do not wish to experience withdrawal bleeding.

5

6 PRE-EXISTING MEDICAL CONDITIONS – HOW SHOULD TREATMENT BE MODIFIED?

6.1 Diabetes.

In the past, considerable concern has surrounded the use of oestrogen replacement treatment in diabetic patients because of the reported adverse effects of oral oestrogen on liver function and, in particular, glucose tolerance (oestrogens increase gluconeogenesis).

However, much of the current dogma has been extrapolated from reports based on the use of oral artificial oestrogens and, whilst artificial oestrogens are diabetogenic, there is no evidence that postmenopausal oestrogen replacement adversely affects carbohydrate metabolism. There is, therefore, no reason to withhold treatment in these women.

Once treatment has begun, glycaemic control should be carefully monitored since progestogens have an anti-insulin effect, and the insulin dose may need to be adjusted to maintain appropriate control (Figure 28). Once the insulin dose has been effectively titrated, and provided no further changes are made to treatment, there is no reason to suppose that the patient should not remain stable.

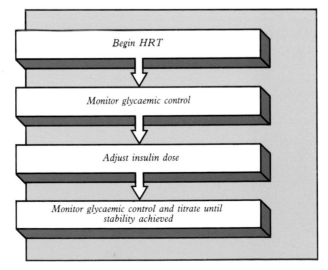

Figure 28. Management of the diabetic patient on HRT.

In view of the increased risk of cardiovascular disease in all diabetic patients, and the "cardioprotective" effect of oestrogens, it could be argued that replacement treatment is essential for this group of patients. The use of progestogens is also of importance since diabetic patients are also at increased risk of endometrial cancer.[105]

McFarland *et al*[106] have shown that in women with angiographically confirmed ischaemic heart disease oestrogens have a protective effect that, in multivariate analysis, is maintained despite diabetes. A similar finding was reached by Paganini-Hill *et al* in their analysis of the effects of oestrogen on stroke.[21]

6.2 Cardiovascular disease.

Re-analysis of various cohort studies has confirmed the overwhelming consensus that oestrogen replacement treatment modifies cardiovasular risk beneficially and is "cardioprotective".[20] This protective action is believed to be mediated partially by beneficial changes in cholesterol levels.

The menopause is associated with a change in the lipoprotein pattern which is not reflected in men of similar age. Total and LDL cholesterol levels rise whilst HDL and VLDL levels fall (Figure 29).[107] Oestrogen treatment reverses this pattern, as shown by the study of Barnes *et al*,[108] in women taking conjugated oestrogens. This is because oestrogens increase HDL and reduce LDL.

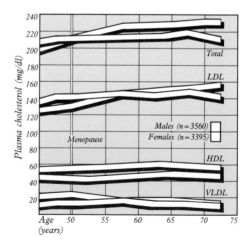

Figure 29. Mean plasma total cholesterol, LDL, HDL and VLDL cholesterol in white North American populations (Lipid Research Clinics Prevalence Study).[107]

A recent review has stated that most prospective studies show at least a 50 per cent reduction in coronary heart disease and related mortality with oestrogen use.[23]

The risk of dying from a myocardial infarction is dramatically reduced in women on oestrogen treatment.[17] A 50 per cent reduction in mortality was reported in women treated with 0.625 mg of conjugated oestrogen when compared with non-treated women.

Thus, once investigations have been performed and the absence of intrinsic hypercoagulability has been confirmed, there is no reason to withhold HRT from patients who have suffered a previous myocardial infarction.

Similarly, oestrogen replacement also produces a 50 per cent reduction in death rate due to stroke.[21] Thus, HRT should not be withheld from patients although the same caveats as above apply.

However, it should be borne in mind that all of the above epidemiological evidence has been generated in the USA where unopposed oestrogen treatment is used widely. Thus, the effect of the addition of a progestogen on such statistics must be considered.

It has been suggested that progestogen addition may attenuate oestrogenic effects,[14] but to date there are no studies to support this statement. Indeed, it is clear that norethisterone 1 mg,[109] or norgestrel 150 μg[110] or dydrogesterone 10-20 mg do not adversely affect the lipid pattern in conventional cyclic opposed regimens (Figure 30).

6

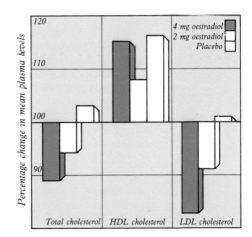

Figure 30. The effect of HRT on lipid profiles. When compared with placebo beneficial changes are seen in total cholesterol, HDL and LDL cholesterol levels from pre-treatment baseline following one year of cyclic opposed treatment: placebo, oestradiol 2 mg and norethisterone acetate 1 mg or oestradiol 4 mg and norethisterone acetate 1mg.[25]

6.3 Previous thromboembolism.

For historical reasons data sheets for the majority of currently available HRT preparations state that previous thromboembolism is a contra-indication to treatment. However, the rationale for this, and the objection to prescribing exogenous replacement oestrogens in such patients, is based upon experience with the contraceptive pill, i.e. upon the theoretical evidence that certain artificial oestrogens have a profound thrombogenic potential in modifying clotting factors and in reducing circulating natural antithrombotic factors such as antithrombin III and plasminogen.

A review by Upton confirms that the natural oestrogens used in HRT cause less thrombogenic disturbance than their artificial counterparts.[46] Indeed, controversy exists over whether natural oestrogens have any clinically significant effect on fibrinolysis and coagulation. To date, no one has demonstrated an increase in thromboembolic risk with oestrogen replacement treatment.

When considering the management of such patients it is useful to distinguish between those in whom a previous thromboembolic episode has resulted from a provoking incident, such as surgery or prolonged bed rest, and those in whom an intrinsic prothrombotic tendency is evident (Figure 31). Only in the latter category is it essential to investigate clotting factor status before HRT may be prescribed — oestrogen use is contra-indicated only in those in whom inherited hypercoagulability is apparent.

Those women who develop thromboembolism in pregnancy or when on the contraceptive pill should be investigated for conditions such as antithrombin III or protein C deficiency which are prothrombotic, rather than assuming that they have demonstrated an abnormal sensitivity to oestrogens.

Patient type	Investigation advised before HRT
Previous DVT provoked by surgery	None
Previous DVT provoked by prolonged bed rest	None
Thromboembolism during pregnancy or whilst taking the contraceptive pill	Screen for intrinsic prothrombotic tendency, antithrombin III or protein C deficiency, abnormal clotting factor status, fibrinogen/platelet malfunction

Figure 31. Management of the patient with a previous thromboembolism.

Additionally, it is important to consider the time interval that has elapsed since the thromboembolic event, and whether there is radiological evidence to support the diagnosis. In the past, many diagnoses of thromboembolism were accepted without objective evidence, whereas it is now clear that venography or ventilation perfusion scanning is needed before confirmation of the diagnosis. Clinical evidence is only accurate in 50 per cent of cases.[111]

It is generally accepted that in patients with previous thrombotic disease oestrogen implants, transvaginal creams or transdermal oestrogen are preferred to the oral route. Parenteral routes enable oestrogen to pass directly into the systemic circulation, thus avoiding the liver where most of the factors involved in fibrinolysis and coagulation are synthesized.

6.4 Epilepsy.

With the exception of sodium valproate, antiepileptic drugs enhance the metabolism of oestrogen by increasing hepatic glucuronidation. Oestrogen glucuronides are rapidly excreted by the kidney and result in low plasma levels of oestrogen. This is well-illustrated by the low plasma oestradiol levels achieved following oral administration of conjugated oestrogens in a woman taking phenytoin (Figure 32).

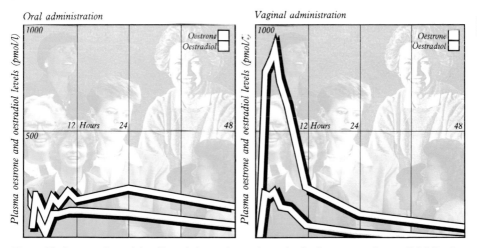

Figure 32. *A comparison of the effect of phenytoin on plasma levels of oestrone and oestradiol following oral or vaginal administration of conjugated equine oestrogen (1.25 mg).[72]*

For patients receiving antiepileptic medication who also require oestrogen treatment the choice is either to use sodium valproate with an oral oestrogen or to use another antiepileptic drug with a parenteral oestrogen preparation.

6.5 Breast cancer.

Because certain breast cancers have been shown to be oestrogen-responsive, reservations exist with regard to the treatment of such patients with HRT. However, there is no data to substantiate the view that HRT increases the risk of metastases, or to demonstrate that patients with malignant breast disease have a reduced survival if they are prescribed oestrogen treatment.

Progestogens are used in the treatment of breast carcinoma; there is therefore no reason to deny progestogen-only treatment, which may be useful in the relief of menopausal symptoms such as flushes and night sweats[99] and, in addition, may conserve bone mass,[97] in these patients. However, it should be remembered that such treatment will not improve vaginal or urinary symptoms.

Where severe menopausal symptoms seriously affect quality of life the patient should be referred to a specialist clinic where oestrogen can be administered under close supervision.

6.6 Endometrial cancer.

Most cases of endometrial cancer, almost 80 per cent in one series,[112] are Stage I tumours with no metastatic disease. Management should therefore be on an individual basis dependent upon the extent of invasion of the myometrium, its histological grading and surgical confirmation that there is no cervical or extrauterine involvement.

In addition, reversal of adenomatous and atypical hyperplasia follows cyclical progestogen administration.[113] No increase in the risk of recurrence has been demonstrated with HRT; rather, in a study of patients with Stage I carcinoma, disease-free survival appeared to be prolonged by treatment (Figure 33).[114]

Figure 33. *Effect of oestrogen treatment on survival following Stage I endometrial carcinoma. Six-year survival in 221 women at the Duke University Medical Center between 1975 and 1980. Oestrogen treatment improved survival.*[114]

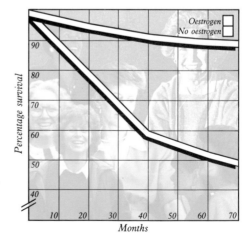

56

6.7 Otosclerosis.

Otosclerosis is a rare condition which has been shown to deteriorate during pregnancy and this observation has been extrapolated to the use of exogenous oestrogens. However, to date, there is no data to demonstrate that otosclerosis deteriorates in patients on HRT.

6.8 Other gynaecological cancers.

There is no evidence that oestrogen plays any role in vaginal, ovarian or cervical cancer, or that HRT increases the risk of these diseases occurring.[115]

Thus, HRT should not be denied to patients in whom these diseases have been, or are being, effectively treated.

6.9 Gallstones.

It is well recognized that both oral artificial oestrogens and oral natural oestrogens increase the risk of gallstones. Whilst this is rare, oral oestrogens should be used with care in patients with gallstones.

As yet, no data exists on the use of transdermal oestrogens in such patients although this route of administration may be advantageous; oestrogens delivered in this way avoid first pass hepatic metabolism and have fewer adverse metabolic effects.[75]

6.10 The woman who smokes.

Smoking is a well-established risk factor for myocardial infarction and stroke. Although oral contraceptive use appears to increase this hazard there is no evidence of such risk enhancement with HRT. The patient should be encouraged to give up smoking and the other cardiovascular risk factors, such as hypertension, should be investigated and treated accordingly. Otherwise there is no reason to treat this group of patients differently from other menopausal women. It is interesting to note that in this group of women oestrogen appears to have the same cardiovascular protective effect against heart attack and stroke as in non-smokers.[17,21,106]

THE BREAST AND HRT

7.1 How should anxiety over the risk of breast cancer be approached?

The effects of oestrogen replacement treatment on the long-term risk of breast cancer remain controversial and no consensus exists at present.

Although numerous epidemiological studies have investigated the relationship between HRT and breast cancer risk many of these are flawed methodologically — failing to take into account important factors which influence breast cancer risk, such as age at menarche, age at menopause and length of treatment. Thus, the results are conflicting. Six large, well-controlled, modern studies have been published and all have shown a lack of adverse effect with short-term use of up to seven years.[116-121]

The potential anxiety about HRT and breast cancer is confined to long-term use for eight years or more. Four studies[55,116,117,120] show long-term effects with, for example, a 1.47 times increase in risk after 20 years of use.[116]

Conversely, three studies[118-120] showed no such effect. None of these studies contain enough patients with long-term use to have sufficient statistical power to answer this question reliably.

For those patients considering long-term treatment over a 10-20 year period careful counselling is required to enable them to make a rational decision between the benefits of treatment and the possible, but not proven, increased breast cancer risk.

Interestingly, there is evidence to suggest that women who develop breast cancer whilst on treatment may have a better prognosis.[122,123] This is shown in Figure 34, which compares survival in oestrogen users and non-users in different age groups postmenopausally.

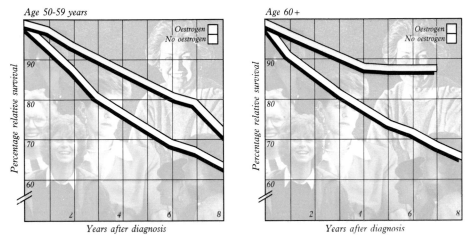

Figure 34. Effect of oestrogen use on relative survival with breast cancer in two menopausal age groups. The relative survival is shown for age 50-59 and 60+ years. Oestrogen users have a significantly lower mortality at 50-59 years (p=0.006) and 60+ years (p=0.004) than non-users.[123]

7.2 How should previous benign breast disease and HRT be approached?

Benign breast disease is not an accepted contra-indication to HRT. The epidemiological evidence is conflicting as to whether prior benign disease confers an increased risk of breast cancer, irrespective of whether oestrogens are used or not.

Brinton's study for the National Cancer Institute[116] suggested a positive association, but Dupont et al, in a large follow-up of women with positive breast biopsies, found that the effect was limited to proliferative or atypical histology with otherwise no risk increase.[124]

Bergkvist et al[123] found a borderline significance for prior positive breast biopsy and breast cancer risk, and pointed out that women with prior positive breast biopsy were more likely to have received oestrogens and that this may be a confounding feature.

The largest study to look at the association between prior positive breast biopsy and oestrogen treatment is that of Dupont et al.[124] This showed that benign breast disease and oestrogen treatment had no overall effect on breast cancer risk and, importantly, showed that oestrogen use in women with potentially more serious abnormalities, such as atypical breast hyperplasia or proliferative disease, reduced the risk of cancer (Table 11). The table shows the risk ratios in these groups. The most logical conclusion is, therefore, that benign breast disease is not a contra-indication to treatment.

Table 11 - EFFECT OF OESTROGENS ON BREAST CANCER RISK IN WOMEN WITH PRIOR BREAST BIOPSY

	Cancer risk (95 per cent confidence intervals)	
Breast histology	No oestrogen	Oestrogen-treated
Not proliferative	0.91 (0.49-1.7)	0.69 (0.40-1.2)
Proliferative without atypia	1.9 (1.48-2.8)	0.92 (0.61-1.4)
Atypical hyperplasia	4.5 (2.5-8.1)	3.0 (1.6-5.5)

Taken from Dupont et al.[124] N.B. Confidence intervals overlapping 1 indicate non-significance.

7.3 How should previous malignant disease and HRT be approached?

Conventional wisdom from both surgeons and oncologists alike is that the use of oestrogen treatment in a woman who has had active recent breast cancer is potentially hazardous.

Only anecdotal data exists to show an increased risk of metastasis with oestrogen treatment but, nevertheless, this view remains widely held. This should not be extrapolated to include all hormone treatments, since menopausal symptoms may be adequately relieved by progestogens alone. The use of vaginal oestriol cream or a 0.025mg vaginal oestradiol tablet has been shown to have no systemic actions.

It should also be remembered that there is no data to support the view that breast cancer is an absolute contra-indication to the use of oestrogen in these patients. Careful counselling and rigorous monitoring are required before oestrogen treatment can be considered, but this may be acceptable to patients who have severe impairment of their quality of life.

In patients in whom metastatic disease is widespread, and whose life expectancy is months rather than years, quality of life is of extreme importance and there is little reason to deny HRT to these women.

7.4 How should patients with a family history of breast disease be treated?

The epidemiological data is at variance regarding risk factors, with no firm evidence that women with a family history of breast cancer are at increased risk when receiving oestrogen replacement treatment. In such patients there is no reason not to prescribe combined sequential treatment.

7.5 How should breast abnormalities detected during treatment be managed?

There is no evidence to suggest that HRT increases the frequency of breast abnormalities although the routine mammographic screening of these patients and annual breast examinations may increase the incidence of detection.

In patients in whom abnormality is detected there is no reason to withdraw treatment until a diagnosis has been confirmed and the implications of this have been discussed thoroughly with the patient.

Malignancy
In the case of malignancy it is often appropriate to withdraw systemic oestrogens; however, treatment should be tailed off over several months to minimize the recurrence of symptoms and should not be withdrawn abruptly. Alternative strategies should be discussed with the patient and other treatment instituted where applicable.

Fibrocystic disease
Benign breast conditions, such as cysts or general nodularity, will occur in a small proportion of women on HRT just as they do in premenopausal women. HRT is not associated with an increased incidence of malignancy in these patients[124] (see Table 11, Section 7.2) so patients should be strongly reassured. If the breast condition is associated with pain then modification of either the oestrogen or the progestogen dose, usually a reduction, is advisable.

Oestrogen-related symptoms will occur throughout the treatment cycle, whereas progestogen-related symptoms will be limited to the premenstrual phase. In very occasional cases oestrogen will have to be avoided and progestogen-only treatment used with vaginal oestriol or low-dose vaginal oestradiol.

Mammographic abnormalities

These may be cystic, solid or show various patterns of calcification. Treatment should not be withdrawn until a positive diagnosis has been established. The management will not alter because of HRT; thus, evaluation of cysts and solid lesions will involve either further imaging with mammography, ultrasound and needle aspiration or, occasionally, excision biopsy.

Calcification may be macro- or microcalcification; the former is always benign but the latter requires careful evaluation. The radiologist reading the mammogram will advise whether it is suspicious and requires localization and biopsy, benign but requires no action, or possibly suspicious requiring follow-up mammography to look for signs of change in the calcification which, if present, would indicate a need for biopsy.

7

8 | LONG-TERM TREATMENT

8.1 What are the frequency and type of long-term symptoms?

Flushes and urogenital symptoms occur in a significant number of women for up to 25 years after ovarian failure (Figure 35).

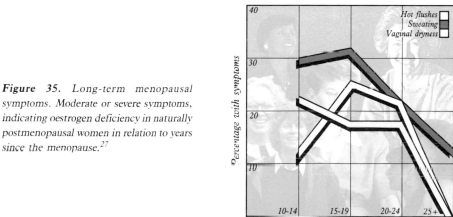

Figure 35. Long-term menopausal symptoms. Moderate or severe symptoms, indicating oestrogen deficiency in naturally postmenopausal women in relation to years since the menopause.[27]

Similar findings on symptom duration were reported by Thompson *et al,*[125] and McKinlay and Jefferys,[3] with 25 per cent of women experiencing flushes for more than five years. This suggests that for the treatment of symptoms alone more women would benefit from long-term treatment than has hitherto been medically recognized.

Since there is no way of predicting which women will suffer in the long-term, it is the woman herself who will necessarily dictate treatment duration. Interestingly, a recent survey of women in Sweden found that 48 per cent of women wished to have life-long treatment.[4] Medical opinion will have to take these attitudes into consideration when planning management.

8.2 How should long-term treatment differ?

There is no reason for long-term treatment to differ in any way from that prescribed for a short duration; it is now recommended that cyclic opposed treatment should be prescribed for all women with an intact uterus, irrespective of the duration of treatment, since the adverse effects of cyclic unopposed oestrogens are well-established (see Sections 3.5 and 3.6).

The importance of a combined regimen is even greater when treatment is to be used long-term, as shown by the increased rates of bleeding, endometrial abnormality and hysterectomy with increasing duration of use of unopposed oestrogen.[54,56]

As discussed elsewhere (see Section 3.5), the dose of oestrogen should be sufficient to relieve symptoms completely. Older women may achieve symptom relief with smaller doses of oestrogen, just as doses of all drugs may need to be reduced with age to allow for reduced metabolism and excretion.

It is important, however, to remember that protection against osteoporosis and cardiovascular disease may be lost with very low doses of oestrogen and the treatment tailored accordingly (see Section 8.3).

8.3 Should HRT be prescribed for osteoporosis?

Osteoporosis is characterized by a reduction in both the amount and strength of bone tissue and leads to an abnormal susceptibility to fracture. It is a major cause of morbidity and mortality in postmenopausal women.[126] This is because accelerated bone loss occurs as a result of oestrogen deficiency and the resultant osteopenia leads to fractures.

The incidence of Colles' fracture and of vertebral fracture increases soon after the menopause (Figure 36), whereas the incidence of hip fracture increases more slowly with age until approximately age 70 when the incidence increases significantly.

The cumulative life-time risk at 50 years of age for either Colles' fracture or hip fracture in women is 15 per cent.[126]

It has been estimated that 50 per cent of women will have an osteoporotic fracture during their lifetime.[127] In reality the prevalence of vertebral fractures cannot be reliably assessed since they do not result in admission to hospital or specific treatments, and all statements about their prevalence must remain purely estimates. Surveys of women give an approximate incidence of vertebral fracture of 25 per cent at age 65.[128] More accurate data is available for femoral neck fracture and in England and Wales this occurs in 12 per cent of women under 85 years of age.[129]

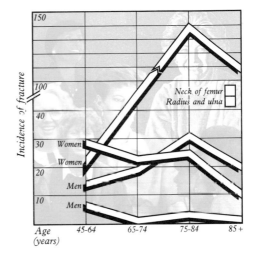

Figure 36. Differences in fracture incidence between men and women. In the years 45-75 the incidence of femoral neck fractures increases in women. The incidence of femoral neck fractures in women is dramatically greater than in men due to the influence of oesteoporosis (Data from Office of Health Economics).

Approximately 20 per cent of women who sustain a fractured neck of femur will die as a direct result of their injury.[130] Other consequences of hip fracture are also severe. In 1985 the average length of hospital stay for hip fracture was 29.8 days.

Those women who do survive hip fracture often suffer permanent disability and, where previously independent, remain in long-term care. Because of this doctors who are treating postmenopausal women should ask themselves, "Is this woman at risk of osteoporosis?" and "Is the treatment prescribed providing adequate skeletal protection?"

The key to the effective management of osteoporosis is prevention rather than treatment. This is because it is difficult to restore mineral and collagen content once osteoporosis has started. The issues are, therefore, how to identify those women who are 'at risk' and what preventive treatment should be provided.

Not all postmenopausal women will develop osteoporosis — other factors, such as peak bone mass and racial origin, are important in this respect but not fully understood. Thus, without access to a bone densitometer the detection of osteoporosis is difficult.

Bone density measurements of the spine and femur can identify not only established osteoporosis but also low initial bone density at the time of menopause and, if used for serial measurements, the rate of bone loss. Low initial bone density, rapid bone loss during the menopause and established osteoporosis all represent significant risks for osteoporotic fracture and are reason enough to prescribe long-term HRT.

When bone densitometry is not available the option of prophylaxis should not be ignored; however, the doctor must rely on the poorly predictive associations of osteoporosis such as family history, low body mass, smoking, high alcohol and low calcium intake.[131]

In addition, there are two groups of women who are at particular risk. These are women taking oral corticosteroids who may develop a Cushing-type osteoporosis, and those with premature ovarian failure in whom bone loss will begin at a young age and continue for a longer period of time than in the average woman.

Oestrogens,[132] progestogen[132] and calcitonin will all successfully prevent bone loss. The role of calcium is disputed[133,134] and the effectiveness of sodium etidronate in preventing bone loss has, so far, been shown by only two studies in patients with established osteoporosis.[103,104]

Oestrogens remain the first-line approach because they are safe, effective and inexpensive. The dose of oestrogen that is required to protect the skeleton and to prevent fractures in a given population is 0.625 mg conjugated equine oestrogen[12] or 2 mg oestradiol (Figure 37).

8

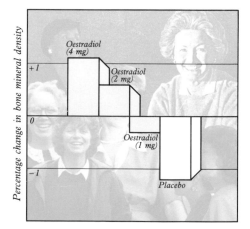

Figure 37. Dose of oestrogen needed for skeletal protection against osteoporosis. Serial bone densitometry in women on different 17β-oestradiol doses allows calculation of positive or negative balance. Whereas 1 mg 17β-oestradiol and placebo are associated with bone loss, 2 mg and 4 mg are associated with an increase in the mean bone mass after six months of treatment with cyclic opposed treatment containing 17β-oestradiol, oestriol and norethisterone.[135]

However, these doses will not protect all of the population[61,136] and larger doses may be needed for some women. Identifying which women will require higher doses has so far proved difficult,[137] but certainly the use of minimal doses of oestrogen should be avoided where preservation of the skeleton is a key objective of treatment.

Where combined sequential treatment is necessary 19-nortestosterone-derived progestogens are thought to have a greater effect on bone mass than progesterone or 17β-hydroxyprogesterone derivatives (Figure 38).[132]

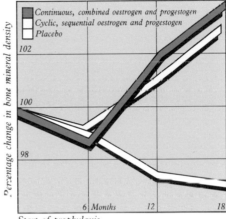

Figure 38. *Percentage change in lumbar spine bone mineral density with sequential or continuous combined oestrogen and progestogen in menopausal women compared with placebo. Bone mineral density changes over 18 months are shown.[138]*

If bone densitometry is available it is prudent to review those patients who are receiving treatment to ensure that bone loss has been arrested. It is not clear, at present, how much bone can be put back when there is established osteoporosis.[100,138–140]

Recent studies suggest that increments of two to three per cent can be achieved over a two-year period[39,103] with unopposed oestrogen, oestrogen combined with progestogen and also sodium etidronate.[103,104] Whether these improvements continue to increase with time has yet to be studied.

There is strong evidence that HRT given for a five to ten year period can prevent osteoporosis and treatment should not be denied to those women who are judged to be 'at risk'.[139] It is important to begin treatment as soon after the menopause as possible.

9 CONTRACEPTION

9.1 When can contraception be stopped safely?

The assessment of fertility around the time of the menopause is difficult since it is clearly impossible to study fertility at this age when unwanted conception would be a particular disadvantage. Diagnosis of menopause and, therefore, the final cessation of fertility is, by definition, retrospective and advice, which is based on certain assumptions, should be cautious.

Whilst it is well-documented that anovulatory cycles in the over 40 age group increase with age some women continue to menstruate regularly and are likely to be fertile. One particular study claims that 95 per cent of women over 40 years of age who reported no change in menstrual pattern ovulated in every cycle, whilst only 34 per cent of those with oligomenorrhoea ovulated consistently (Figure 39).[141]

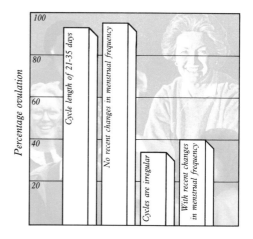

Figure 39. *The relationship of the pattern of menstrual cycle to ovulation. Women were studied in three consecutive cycles. Those with regular cycles or a cycle length of 21-25 days had a 95 and 93 per cent incidence of ovulation respectively. Conversely, irregular cycles or recent menstrual change were associated with only 34 and 40 per cent ovulation respectively.[141]*

Although it is clear that not every ovulation will be fertile, and that increasing periods of amenorrhoea coupled with less frequent intercourse mean that conception is less likely to occur in this age group, 50 per cent of women under the age of 50 with amenorrhoea for six months will have one further ovulation at least.[141] Thus, effective contraception is vital during this period to minimize anxieties over an unwanted pregnancy.

The rapid fluctuations in ovarian function at this time produce on the one hand menopausal symptoms, elevated FSH and amenorrhoea, and on the other re-establishment of menstruation, declining FSH and symptom resolution. Accordingly, a single FSH measurement showing elevated serum levels should not be seen as an indicator for withdrawal of contraception since ovulation can occur in spite of raised gonadotrophin levels. It is therefore prudent to advise maintaining contraception until amenorrhoea has been established for one full year.

Those women who are using hormonal methods of contraception will have good protection and it is probably reasonable to begin HRT at the age of 50.

9.2 Is HRT contraceptive?

The contraceptive efficacy of the natural oestrogens used in most forms of HRT has yet to be adequately established and, in perimenopausal women particularly, should not be relied upon.

The average dose of oestrogen in HRT is equivalent to 10 μg of the commonly used artificial contraceptive oestrogen, ethinyl oestradiol. Whilst this is significantly lower than the doses that are used in the contraceptive pill to suppress ovarian function, it should be remembered that such high doses are designed primarily for the younger woman with full ovarian function and not for those women with declining levels of ovarian hormones. Thus, there is potential for a contraceptive effect with standard HRT doses.

High doses of natural oestrogens can suppress ovulation. A daily oral dose of 7.5 mg conjugated equine oestrogen, at least six times higher than the normal replacement dose, will suppress ovarian function but may affect the thrombogenic potential of standard HRT.[142]

In theory, at least, continuous combined HRT regimens should be contraceptive since they are designed to achieve amenorrhoea and endometrial atrophy.[143] At present there is little data to substantiate this; one disadvantage of such an approach is that amenorrhoea in a premenopausal woman may be a source of anxiety and necessitate withdrawal from treatment if the patient is not appropriately counselled.

In a study of the contraceptive effects of 100 mg oestradiol implants in premenopausal women, 50 per cent showed follicular development during the first three cycles, with evidence of follicular rupture and luteinization in a small proportion up to that time (Figure 40).[144]

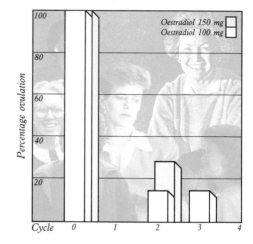

Figure 40. Ovulation in patients treated with 17β-oestradiol implants. Ovulation frequency (%) is shown for the months after implantation of two doses of oestrogen, 100 mg or 150 mg. There was no ovulation after two months with 150 mg or three months with 100 mg.[51]

After six months of treatment ovulation was suppressed in all women, demonstrating clear contraceptive effects. The introduction of a second implant ensured continuing ovarian suppression. The implant should be inserted early in the menstrual cycle and the recommended maintenance dose is 50 mg oestradiol every six months, eventually reducing to 25 mg oestradiol every six months.

More recently, combined sequential formulations containing oestradiol valerate with either cyproterone acetate or norethisterone have been studied for their contraceptive effect in women over 35 years of age.[145] In the course of one year no pregnancies were reported, but serum progesterone measurements suggested that one ovulation had occurred in the cyproterone acetate group and 11 in the norethisterone group, with breakthrough bleeding in up to 40 per cent of cases.

A preliminary study of transdermal oestrogen in 10 premenopausal volunteers showed that the use of 200 μg transdermal oestradiol patches every three days suppressed follicular activity and ovulation in all cases by the second month of treatment, suggesting a contraceptive potential.[146]

In summary, therefore, the only HRT regimen with certain contraceptive effect is the use of high-dose oestradiol implants. Although oral and transdermal regimens will undoubtedly suppress an already diminished fertility, sporadic ovulation still occurs and women need to continue contraception until the frequency of ovulation diminishes. This is arbitrarily taken to be 12 months from clinical evidence of the menopause.

9.3 What contraceptive choices are available?

There is increasing awareness that women over 40 require both effective contraception and HRT for menopausal symptom relief.

Effectively, the methods of contraception in this age group do not differ from those available to the younger woman. In fact, declining fertility in these women means that many of these methods are relatively more effective.

Most experts now agree that the modern, low dose oestrogen/progestogen pill can be used up to the age of 45 in those women who are not smokers and who have no cardiovascular risk factors. The development of new, non-oral forms of delivery may increase the safety of such treatment in terms of the cardiovascular risk in older women.

For those women with cardiovascular risk factors the progestogen-only pill represents an alternative that can be used until the time of menopause. Progestogen alone can also be administered by a variety of other routes such as depot injection, implant or vaginal ring.

In the older woman the efficacy of barrier and IUCD methods is higher than in young women. Additionally, the contraceptive sponge can be recommended for women with low fertility and those over age 45. Many women, or their partners, will of course have opted for sterilization by this age.

Natural family planning methods are not dependable in the older woman because of hormonal fluctuations and dysfunction.

9

10 PATIENT SYMPTOM QUESTIONNAIRE

Name: _____

NHS no: _____

Are you suffering from:

- [ ] Hot flushes?
- [ ] Night sweats?
- [ ] Loss of memory or concentration?
- [ ] Poor sleep?
- [ ] Dry skin or hair?
- [ ] Problems with teeth or gums?
- [ ] Urinary frequency?
- [ ] Incontinence of urine?
- [ ] Sexual problems e.g.
- [ ] — Reduced sex drive?
- [ ] — Dryness or soreness?
- [ ] — Reduced sexual satisfaction?
- [ ] — Aversion to touching/kissing?
- [ ] Lack of confidence e.g.
- [ ] — Unwillingness to go out?
- [ ] — Fear of entertaining?
- [ ] — Fear of going into supermarket?
- [ ] Depressed or anxious mood?
- [ ] Lethargy/loss of energy/tiredness?
- [ ] Joint or limb pains?

Please tick box

REFERENCES

1. Bungay GT, Vessey MP, McPherson CK. Study of symptoms in middle life with special reference to the menopause. *Br Med J* 1980; **ii**: 181-183.

2. Campbell S, Whitehead MI. Oestrogen therapy and the menopausal syndrome. *Clin Obstet Gynaecol* 1977; **4**: 31-47.

3. McKinlay SM, Jefferys M. The menopausal syndrome. *Br J Prev Soc Med* 1974; **28**: 108-115.

4. Samsioe G, Bryman I, Ivansson E. Some anthropological aspects of the climacteric syndrome. *Acta Obstet Gynecol Scand* 1985; **130 (Suppl)**: 5-7.

5. Coope J, Thomson JM, Poller L. Effects of 'natural oestrogen' replacement therapy on menopausal symptoms and blood-clotting. *Br Med J* 1975; **4**: 139-143.

6. Dennerstein L, Burrows GD, Hyman GJ, Sharpe K. Some clinical effects of oestrogen-progestogen therapy in surgically castrated women. *Maturitas* 1979; **2**: 19-28.

7. Hunt K. Perceived value of treatment among a group of long-term users of hormone replacement therapy. *J R Coll Gen Pract* 1988; **38**: 398-401.

8. Versi E, Cardozo L. Oestrogens and lower urinary tract function. In: Studd JWW, Whitehead MI, eds. *The Menopause.* Oxford: Blackwell Scientific Publications, 1988; 76-84.

9. Clayden JR, Bell JW, Pollard P. Menopausal flushing: double-blind trial of a non-hormonal medication. *Br Med J* 1974; **1**: 409-412.

10. Christiansen C, Christensen MS, Transbol I. Bone mass in postmenopausal women after withdrawal of oestrogen/gestogen replacement therapy. *Lancet* 1981; **1**: 459-461.

11. Munk-Jensen N 1990. Data on file.

12. Gordan GS, Picchi J, Roof BS. Antifracture efficacy of long-term estrogens for osteoporosis. *Trans Assoc Am Physicians* 1973; **86**: 326-332.

13. Paganini-Hill A, Ross RK, Gerkins VR, Henderson BE, Arthur M, Mack T. Menopausal oestrogen therapy and hip fractures. *Ann Intern Med* 1981; **95**: 28-31.

14. Ross RK. Stroke prevention and oestrogen replacement therapy. *Lancet* 1989; **1**: 505.

15. Stevenson JC. Pathogenesis, prevention and treatment of osteoporosis. *Obstet Gynecol* 1990; **75 (Suppl 4)**: 36s-41s.

16. Vessey M, Hunt K. The menopause, hormone replacement therapy and cardiovascular disease: epidemiological aspects. In: Studd JWW, Whitehead MI, eds. *The Menopause.* Oxford: Blackwell Scientific Publications, 1988; 190-196.

17. Ross RK, Paganini-Hill A, Mack TM, Arthur M, Henderson BE. Menopausal oestrogen therapy and protection from death from ischaemic heart disease. *Lancet* 1981; **1**: 858-860.

18. Hunt K, Vessey M, McPherson K, Coleman M. Long-term surveillance of mortality and cancer incidence in women receiving hormone replacement therapy. *Br J Obstet Gynaecol* 1987; **94**: 620-635.

11

19. Hunt K, Vessey M. Long term effects of postmenopausal hormone therapy. *Br J Hosp Med* 1987; **Nov:** 450-459.

20. Consensus Report, Consensus Development Conference, Copenhagen 1990. (In press).

21. Paganini-Hill A, Ross RK, Henderson BE. Postmenopausal oestrogen treatment and stroke: A prospective study. *Br Med J* 1988; **297:** 519-522.

22. Gruchow HW, Anderson AJ, Barboriak JJ, Sobocinski KA. Postmenopausal use of estrogen and occlusion of coronary arteries. *Am Heart J* 1988; **115:** 954-963.

23. Lobo RA. Cardiovascular implications of estrogen replacement therapy. *Obstet Gynecol* 1990; **75 (Suppl 4):** 18s-25s.

24. Hirvonen E, Mälkönen M, Manninen V. Effects of different progestogens on lipoproteins during postmenopausal replacement therapy. *N Engl J Med* 1981; **304:** 560-563.

25. Jensen J, Christiansen C. Dose-response effects on serum lipids and lipoproteins following combined oestrogen-progestogen therapy in post-menopausal women. *Maturitas* 1987; **9:** 259-266.

26. Clarkson TB, Adams MR, Shrively CA, Koritnik DR. Reevaluation of lipid effects on atherosclerosis. *Consensus Development Conference on Progestogens International Proceedings Journal* 1989; **1:** 262-265.

27. Hagstad A, Janson PO. The epidemiology of climacteric symptoms. *Acta Obstet Gynecol Scand* 1986; **134 (Suppl):** 59s-65s.

28. Parrish HM, Carr CA, Hall DG, King TM. Time interval from castration in premenopausal women to development of excessive coronary atherosclerosis. *Am J Obstet Gynecol* 1967; **99:** 155-162.

29. Richelson LS, Wahner HW, Melton LJ III, Riggs BL. Relative contributions of aging and estrogen deficiency to postmenopausal bone loss. *N Engl J Med* 1984; **311:** 1273-1275.

30. Whitehead MI, King RJB, McQueen J, *et al.* Endometrial histology and biochemistry in climacteric women during oestrogen and oestrogen/progestogen therapy. *J R Soc Med* 1979; **72:** 322-327.

31. Whitehead MI, Fraser D. The effects of estrogens and progestagens on the endometrium. Modern approach to treatment. In: *Obstetrics and Gynecology Clinics of North America* 1987; **28:** 299-320.

32. Sturdee DW, Wade-Evans T, Gustafson R, Studd JWW. Endometrial histology of post-menopausal women receiving various regimens of oestrogen therapy. *Br J Obstet Gynaecol* 1977; **84:** 315-316.

33. Sturdee DW, Wade-Evans T, Paterson MEL, Thom M, Studd JWW. Relations between bleeding pattern, endometrial histology and oestrogen treatment in menopausal women. *Br Med J* 1978; **1:** 1575-1577.

34. Studd JWW, Thom MH, Paterson MEL, Wade-Evans T. The prevention and treatment of endometrial pathology in post-menopausal women receiving exogenous oestrogens. In: Pasetto N, Paoletti R, Ambrus JL, eds. *The Menopause and Postmenopause.* Lancaster: MTP Press, 1980; 127-139.

35. Silverberg SG. Hyperplasia and carcinoma of the endometrium. *Semin Diagn Pathol* 1988; **5:** 135-153.

36. Peterson HB, Lee NC, Rubin GL. Genital neoplasia. In: Mishell DR Jr, ed. *Menopause, Physiology and Pharmacology.* Chicago: Year Book Medical Publishers, Inc, 1987; 275-300.

37. Gambrell RD. Sex steroids and cancer. *Obstetrics and Gynecological Clinics of North America* 1987; **14:** 191-206.

11

38. Wren BG. Cost-effectiveness of hormonal replacement therapy. In: Zichella L, Whitehead M, Van Keep PA, eds. *The Climacteric and Beyond*. Carnforth: Parthena Publishing Group, 1988; 55-62.

39. Whitehead MI, Hillard TC, Crook D. The role and use of progestogens. *Obstet Gynecol* 1990; **75 (Suppl 4)**: 59s-79s.

40. Staland B. Continuous treatment with a combination of estrogen and gestagen — a way of avoiding endometrial stimulation. Clinical experiences with Kliogest[R]. *Acta Obstet Gynecol Scand* 1985; **130 (Suppl)**: 29-35.

41. Staland B. Continuous treatment with natural oestrogens and progestogens. A method to avoid endometrial stimulation. *Maturitas* 1981; **3**: 145-156.

42. Mattson L-A, Cullberg G, Samsioe G. Evaluation of a continuous oestrogen - progestogen regimen for climacteric complaints. *Maturitas* 1982; **4**: 95-102.

43. Stern MD. Pharmacology of conjugated oestrogens. *Maturitas* 1982; **4**: 333-339.

44. Mashchak CA, Lobo RA, Dozono-Takano R, *et al.* Comparison of pharmacodynamic properties of various oestrogen formulations. *Am J Obstet Gynecol* 1982; **144**: 511-518.

45. Geola FL, Frumar AM, Tataryn IV, *et al.* Biologic effects of various doses of conjugated equine estrogens in postmenopausal women. *J Clin Endocrinol Metab* 1980; **51**: 620-625.

46. Upton V. Contraception in the woman over forty. In: Studd JWW, Whitehead MI, eds. *The Menopause*. Oxford: Blackwell Scientific Publications, 1988; 289-304.

47. Campbell S, Whitehead MI. Potency and hepato-cellular effects of oestrogens after oral, percutaneous and subcutaneous administration. In: Van Keep PA, Utian W, Vermeulen A, eds. *The Controversial Climacteric*. Manchester: MTP Press, 1982; 103-125.

48. Stumpf PG. Pharmacokinetics of estrogen. *Obstet Gynecol* 1990; **75 (Suppl 4)**: 9s-14s.

49. Owen EJ, Siddle NC, McGarrigle T, Pugh MA. Choosing the optimum dose of oestradiol implant - pharmacokinetics and symptom relief with 25mg oestradiol implantation. *Presented at Br Soc Obstet Gynaecol, London* 1989.

50. Owen EJ, McGarrigle H, Siddle NC. Clinical and pharmacokinetic effects of 25mg oestradiol implants. (In press, 1990).

51. Studd JWW, Magos M. Hormone pellet implantation for the menopause and premenstrual syndrome. *Obstetrics and Gynecology Clinics of North America* 1987; **14**: 229-250.

51a. Cardozo LD. Routes of oestrogen administration. In: Studd JWW, Whitehead MI, eds. *The Menopause*. Oxford: Blackwell Scientific Publications, 1988; 138-145.

52. *Padwick ML, Endacott J, Whitehead MI. Efficacy, acceptability and metabolic effects of transdermal estradiol in the management of postmenopausal women. Am J Obstet Gynecol 1985;* **152**: 1085-1091.

53. Coope J. Why treat the menopause? In: *The Menopause*. London: Royal College of General Practitioners, 1990; 15-23.

54. Persson I, Adami H-O, Bergkvist L, *et al.* Risk of endometrial cancer after treatment with oestrogens alone or in conjunction with progestogens: Results of a prospective study. *Br Med J* 1989; **298**: 147-151.

55. Ross RK, Paganini-Hill A, Gerkins VR, *et al.* A case control study of menopausal estrogen therapy and breast cancer. *JAMA* 1980; **243**: 1635-1639.

56. Ettinger B, Golditch IM, Fredman G. Gynecologic consequences of long term unopposed estrogen replacement therapy. *Maturitas* 1988; **10**: 271-282.

11

57. Gambrell RD. Prevention of endometrial cancer with progestogens. *Maturitas* 1986; **8**: 159-168.

58. Shapiro S, Kelly JP, Rosenberg L, *et al.* Risk of localized and widespread endometrial cancer in relation to recent and discontinued use of conjugated estrogens. *N Engl J Med* 1985; **313**: 969-972.

59. Siddle NC. Psychological effects of different progestogens. In: *Consensus Development Conference on Progestogens International Proceedings Journal* 1989; **1**: 214-217.

60. Varma TR. Effect of long-term therapy with estrogen and progesterone on the endometrium of post-menopausal women. *Acta Obstet Gynecol Scand* 1985; **64**: 41-46.

61. Whitehead MI, Stevenson JC, Fraser D, Schenkel L, Crook D, Stevenson JC. Transdermal administration of oestrogen/progestagen hormone replacement therapy. *Lancet* 1990; **336**: 310-312.

62. Bradley DD, Wingerd J, Petitti DB, Krauss RM, Ramcharan S. Serum high density lipoprotein cholesterol in women using oral contraceptives, estrogens and progestins. *N Engl J Med* 1978; **299**: 17-20.

63. Siddle NC, Young O, Minardi S, King RJB, Whitehead MI. Dose dependent effects of synthetic progestagens on the oestrogenised postmenopausal endometrium. *Acta Obstet Gynecol Scand* 1982; **106 (Suppl)**: 17-22.

64. Whitehead MI, Siddle N, Lane G, *et al.* The pharmacology of progestogens. In: Mishell DR, ed. *Menopause, Physiology and Pharmacology.* Chicago: Year Book Medical Publishers, 1986; 317-334.

65. Siddle NC, Jesinger DK, Whitehead MI, Turner P, Lewis B, Prescott P. The efficacy, safety and acceptability of dydrogesterone when added to postmenopausal oestrogen treatment. Part 1: Effects on plasma lipids, lipoproteins and triglycerides. (In press, 1990).

66. Siddle NC, Jesinger DK, Whitehead MI, Turner P, Lewis B, Prescott P. The efficacy, safety and acceptability of dydrogesterone when added to postmenopausal oestrogen treatment. Part 2: Endometrial, physical and psychological effects. (In press, 1990).

67. Paterson MEL, Wade-Evans T, Sturdee DW, Thom MH, Studd JWW. Endometrial disease after treatment with oestrogens and progestogens in the climacteric. *Br Med J* 1980; **280**: 822-824.

68. Padwick ML, Pryse-Davies J, Whitehead MI. A simple method for determining the optimal dose of progestin in postmenopausal women receiving estrogens. *N Engl J Med* 1986; **315**: 930-934.

69. Lane G, Siddle NC, Ryder TA, Pryse-Davies J, King RJB, Whitehead MI. Effects of dydrogesterone on the oestrogenised postmenopausal endometrium. *Br J Obstet Gynaecol* 1986; **93**: 55-62.

70. Lane G, Siddle NC, Ryder TA, Pryse-Davies J, King RJB, Whitehead MI. Is Provera the ideal progestin to add to postmenopausal estrogen therapy? *Fertil Steril* 1986; **45**: 345-352.

71. Lane G, Siddle NC, Ryder TA, Pryse-Davies J, King RJB, Whitehead MI. Dose-dependent effects of oral progesterone on the oestrogenized postmenopausal endometrium. *Br Med J* 1983; **287**: 1241-1245.

72. Englund DE, Johansson EDB. Plasma levels of oestrone, oestradiol and gonadotrophins in postmenopausal women after oral and vaginal administration of conjugated equine oestrogens (Premarin). *Br J Obstet Gynaecol* 1978; **85**: 957-964.

73. De Lignieres B, Basdevant A, Thomas G, *et al.* Biologic effects of estradiol 17β in postmenopausal women: oral *versus* percutaneous administration. *J Clin Endocrinol Metab* 1986; **62**: 536-541.

74. Larsson-Cohn U, Wallentin L. Sex steroids and lipoproteins. In: Van Herendael H, Van Herendael B, Riphagen FE, Goessens L, Van der Pas H, eds. *The Climacteric: An Update.* Manchester: MTP Press Ltd, 1984; 75-81.

75. Boston Collaborative Drug Surveillance Program. Surgically confirmed cases of gall bladder disease, venous thromboembolism, and breast tumors in relation to post menopausal estrogen therapy. *N Engl J Med* 1974; **290**: 15-18.

76. Campagnoli C, Tousijn LP, Belforte P, Ferruzzi L, Dolfin AM, Morra G. Effects of conjugated equine oestrogens and oestriol on blood clotting, plasma lipids and endometrial proliferation in post-menopausal women. *Maturitas* 1981; **3**: 135-144.

77. Gangar K, Cust M, Whitehead MI. Symptoms of oestrogen deficiency associated with supraphysiological plasma oestradiol concentrations in women with oestradiol implants. *Br Med J* 1989; **299**: 601-602.

78. Davis GF, Winter L. Cumulative irritation study of placebo and transdermal estrogen patches. *Current Therapeutic Research* 1987; **42**: 712-719.

79. Utian W. Transdermal estradiol overall safety profile. *Am J Obstet Gynecol* 1987; **156**: 1335-1338.

80. Magos AL, Brewster E, Singh R, O'Dowd T, Brincat M, Studd JWW. The effects of norethisterone in postmenopausal women on oestrogen replacement therapy: A model for the premenstrual syndrome. *Br J Obstet Gynaecol* 1986; **93**: 1290-1296.

81. Nachtigall LE, Nachtigall RH, Nachtigall RB, Beckman EM. Estrogen replacement therapy II. A prospective study in the relationship to carcinoma and cardiovascular and metabolic problems. *Obstet Gynecol* 1979; **54**. 74-79.

82. Wren BG, Routledge AD. The effect of type and dose of oestrogen on the blood pressure of post-menopausal women. *Maturitas* 1983; **5**: 135-142.

83. Carr BR. Progestogens: Effect on water/salt metabolism and blood pressure. In: *Consensus Development Conference on Progestogens International Proceedings Journal* 1989; **1**: 87-92.

84. Nachtigall LE. Cardiovascular disease and hypertension in older women. In: Gambrell RD, ed. *The Menopause. Obstetrics and Gynecology Clinics of North America* 1987; **14**: 89-105.

85. Amery A, Brixxo P, Clement D, *et al*. Mortality and morbidity results from The European Working Party on Blood Pressure in the Elderly trial. *Lancet* 1985; **2**: 1349-1354.

86. Whitehead MI, Campbell S. Endometrial histology, uterine bleeding and oestrogen levels in menopausal women receiving oestrogen therapy. In: Brush MG, King RJB, Taylor RW, eds. *Endometrial Cancer*. London: Baillière Tindall, 1978; 65-80.

87. Paganini-Hill A, Ross RK, Henderson BE. Endometrial cancer and patterns of use of estrogen replacement therapy: A cohort study. *Br J Cancer* 1989; **59**: 445-447.

88. Acheson ED. Breast cancer screening. *J R Soc Med* 1989; **82**: 455-457.

89. Roberts MM, Alexander FE, Anderson TJ, *et al*. Edinburgh trial of screening for breast cancer: mortality at seven years. *Lancet* 1990; **335**: 241-246.

90. Vandekerckhove D, Dhont M, Serreyn R. Considerations on the output of pituitary gonadotrophins in the perimenopause. In: Van Herendael H, Van Herendael B, Riphagen FE, Goessens L, Van der Pas H, eds. *The Climacteric: An Update*. Manchester: MTP Press Ltd, 1984; 87-99.

91. Ylostalo P, Vartiainene, Stenman VH, Widholm O. Ovarian function during oestrogen-progestin replacement treatment in pre-menopausal women. *Maturitas* 1986; **8**: 19-27.

92. Johansson BW, Kaig L, Kullander S, Lenner H-C, Svanberg L, Astedt B. On some late effects of bilateral oophorectomy in the age range 15-30 years. *Acta Obstet Gynecol Scand* 1975; **54**: 449-461.

11

93. Gordon T, Kannel WB, Hjortland MC, McNamara PM. Menopause and coronary heart disease. The Framingham Study. *Ann Intern Med* 1978; **9:** 157-161.

94. Rosenberg L, Hennekens CH, Rosner B, Belanger C, Rothman KJ, Speizer FE. Early menopause and the risk of myocardial infarction. *Am J Obstet Gynecol* 1981; **139:** 47-51.

95. Weinstein L. Hormone therapy in the patient with surgical menopause. *Obstet Gynecol* 1990; **75 (Suppl 4):** 47s-52s.

96. Siddle NC, Sarrell P, Whitehead MI. The effect of hysterectomy on the age at ovarian failure: identification of a subgroup of women with premature loss of ovarian function and literature review. *Fertil Steril* 1987; **47:** 94-100.

97. Abdalla HI, McKay Hart D, Lindsay R, Leggate I, Hooke A. Prevention of bone mineral loss in postmenopausal women by norethisterone. *Obstet Gynecol* 1985; **66:** 789-792.

98. Paterson MEL. A randomised double-blind crossover trial into the effect of norethisterone on climacteric symptoms and biochemical profiles. *Br J Obstet Gynaecol* 1982; **89:** 464-472.

99. Wesel S. Clinical effects of vaginally applied oestrogens. In: Van Herendael H, Van Herendael B, Riphagen FE, Goessens L, Van der Pas H, eds. *The Climacteric: An Update.* Manchester: MTP Press Ltd, 1984; 141-148.

100. Christiansen C, Riis BJ. 17β-Estradiol and continuous norethisterone: a unique treatment for established osteoporosis in elderly women. *J Clin Endocrinol Metab* 1990; **71:** 836-841.

101. Civitelli R, Agnusdei D, Nardi P, Zacchei F, Avioli LV, Gennari C. Effects of one-year treatment with estrogens on bone mass, intestinal calcium absorption, and 25-hydroxyvitamin D-1α hydroxylase reserve in postmenopausal osteoporosis. *Calcif Tissue Int* 1988; **42:** 77-86.

102. Reginster JY, Denis D, Albert A, *et al.* 1-year controlled randomised trial of prevention of early menopausal bone loss by intranasal calcitonin. *Lancet* 1987; **2:** 1481-1483.

103. Storm T, Thamsborg G, Steiniche T, Genant HK, Sorensen OH. Effect of intermittent cyclical etidronate therapy on bone mass and fracture rate in women with postmenopausal osteoporosis. *N Engl J Med* 1990; **18:** 1265-1271.

104. Watts NB, Harris ST, Genant HK, *et al.* Intermittent cyclical etidronate treatment of postmenopausal osteoporosis. *N Engl J Med* 1990; **323:** 73-99.

105. Wynder EL, Escher GC, Mantel N. An epidemiological investigation of cancer of the endometrium. *Cancer* 1966; **19:** 489-520.

106. McFarland KF, Boniface ME, Hornung CA, Earnhardt W, Humphries JON. Risk factors and noncontraceptive estrogen use in women with and without coronary disease. *Am Heart J* 1989; **117:** 1209-1214.

107. Crook D, Godsland IF, Wynn V. Ovarian hormones and plasma lipoproteins. In: Whitehead MI, Studd JWW, eds. *The Menopause.* Oxford: Blackwell Scientific Publications, 1988; 169-181.

108. Barnes RB, Roy S, Lobo RA. Comparison of lipid and androgen levels after conjugated estrogen or depomedroxyprogesterone acetate treatment in postmenopausal women. *Obstet Gynecol* 1985; **66:** 216-219.

109. Fletcher CD, Farish E, Hart DM, *et al.* Effect on lipoproteins of Trisequens, a combined hormone preparation. *Maturitas* 1984; **6:** 279-283.

110. Fletcher CD, Farish E, Dagen MM, Hart DM. A comparison of the effects on lipoproteins of two progestogens used during cyclical hormone replacement therapy. *Maturitas* 1987; **9:** 253-258.

11

78

111. Whitehouse G. Radiological diagnosis of deep vein thrombosis. *Br Med J* 1987; **295**: 801-802.

112. Kneale BLG. Adjunctive and therapeutic progestins in endometrial cancer. *Clin Obstet Gynaecol* 1986; **13**: 789-807.

113. Thom H, White PJ, Williams RM, *et al*. Prevention and treatment of endometrial disease in climacteric women receiving oestrogen therapy. *Lancet* 1979; **2**: 455-457.

114. Creasman WT, Henderson D, Hinshaw W, Clarke-Pearson DL. Estrogen replacement therapy in the patient treated for endometrial cancer. *Obstet Gynecol* 1986; **67**: 326-330.

115. Whitehead MI, Fraser D. Controversies concerning the safety of estrogen replacement therapy. *Am J Obstet Gynecol* 1987; **156**: 1313-1322.

116. Brinton LA, Hoover RN, Fraumeni JF. Menopausal oestrogens and breast cancer risk: An expanded case-control study. *Br J Cancer* 1986; **54**: 825-832.

117. Hiatt RA, Bawol R, Friedman GD, Hoover R. Exogenous estrogen and breast cancer after bilateral oophorectomy. *Cancer* 1984; **54**: 139-144.

118. Kelsey JL, Fischer DB, Holfold TR, *et al*. Exogenous estrogens and other factors in the epidemiology of breast cancer. *J Natl Cancer Inst* 1981; **67**: 327-333.

119. Kaufman DW, Miller DR, Rosenberg L, *et al*. Noncontraceptive estrogen use and the risk of breast cancer. *JAMA* 1984; **252**: 63-67.

120. Wingo PA, Layde PM, Lee NC, *et al*. The risk of breast cancer in postmenopausal women who have used estrogen replacement therapy. *JAMA* 1987; **257**: 209-215.

121. Bergkvist L, Adami HO, Persson I, Hoover R, Schairer C. The risk of breast cancer after estrogen and estrogen/progestin replacement. *N Engl J Med* 1989; **321**: 293-297.

122. Gambrell RD. Proposal to decrease risk and improve the prognosis of breast cancer. *Am J Obstet Gynecol* 1984; **150**: 119-132.

123. Bergkvist L, Adami HO, Persson I, Bergström R, Krusemo UB. Prognosis after breast cancer diagnosis in women exposed to estrogen and estrogen-progestogen replacement therapy. *Am J Epidemiol* 1989; **130**: 221-228.

124. Dupont WD, Page DL, Rogers LW, Parl FF. Influence of exogenous estrogens, proliferative breast disease, and other variables on breast cancer risk. *Cancer* 1989; **63**: 948-957.

125. Thompson B, Hart SA, Durno D. Menopausal age and symptomatology in a general practice. *J Biosoc Sci* 1975; **5**: 71-82.

126. Cummings SR, Kelsey JL, Nevitt MC, O'Dowd KJ. Epidemiology of osteoporosis and osteoporotic fractures. *Epidemiol Rev* 1985; **7**: 178-207.

127. Jensen GF, Christiansen C, Boesen J, Hegedus V, Transbol I. Epidemiology of postmenopausal spinal and long bone fractures: A unifying approach to postmenopausal osteoporosis. *Clin Orthop* 1982; **166**: 75-81.

128. Heaney RP. Estrogens and postmenopausal osteoporosis. *Clin Obstet Gynaecol* 1976; **19**: 791-803.

129. Royal College of Physicians. *Fractured Neck of Femur. Prevention and Management*. London: Royal College of Physicians, 1989.

130. Fenton Lewis A. Fracture of neck of femur: changing incidence. *Br Med J* 1981; **283**: 1217-1219.

131. Stevenson JC, Lees B, Devonport M, Cust MP, Gangar KF, Whitehead MI. Determinants of bone density in normal women: risk factors for future osteoporosis? *Br Med J* 1989; **298**: 924-928.

11

132. Lindsay R, Aitken JM, Hart DM, Purdie D. The effect of ovarian sex steroids on bone mineral status in the oophorectomised rat and in the human. *Postgrad Med J* 1978; **54 (Suppl 2):** 50-58.

133. Kanis JA, Passmore R. Calcium supplementation of the diet II. *Br Med J* 1989; **298:** 205-208.

134. Nordin C, Heaney RP. Calcium supplementation of the diet: justified by present evidence. *Br Med J* 1990; **300:** 1056-1060.

135. Christensen MS, Hagen C, Christiansen C, Transbol I. Dose-response evaulation of cyclic estrogen/gestagen in postmenopausal women: Placebo-controlled trial of its gynecologic and metabolic actions. *Am J Obstet Gynecol* 1982; **144:** 873-879.

136. Savvas M, Studd JS. Skeletal effects of oral oestrogen compared with subcutaneous oestrogen and testosterone in postmenopausal women. *Br Med J* 1989; **297:** 331-333.

137. Stevenson JC, Cust MP, Gangar KF, Hillard TC, Lees B, Whitehead MI. Effects of transdermal versus oral hormone replacement therapy on bone density in spine and proximal femur in postmenopausal women. *Lancet* 1990; **335:** 265-269.

138. Munk-Jensen N, Nielsen SP, Obel EB, Eriksen PB. Reversal of postmenopausal vertebral bone loss by oestrogen and progestagen: a double blind placebo controlled study. *Br Med J* 1988; **296:** 1150-1152.

139. Consensus Development Conference. Prophylaxis and treatment of osteoporosis. *Br Med J* 1987; **295:** 914-915.

140. Lindsay R, Tohme JF. Estrogen treatment of patients with established postmenopausal osteoporosis. *Obstet Gynecol* 1990; **76:** 290-295.

141. Metcalf MG. Incidence of ovulatory cycles in women approaching the menopause. *J Biosoc Sci* 1979; **11:** 39-48.

142. Kubba A. Contraception in the climacteric. In: *Focus - The Menopause.* London: Medicom Ltd, 1990; 27-32.

143. Magos AL, Brincat M, Studd JWW, Wardle TJ, Schlesinger P, O'Dowd T. Amenorrhea and endometrial atrophy with continuous oral estrogen and progestogen therapy in postmenopausal women. *Obstet Gynecol* 1985; **65:** 496-499.

144. Magos AL, Collins WP, Studd JWW. Effects of subcutaneous oestradiol implants on ovarian activity. *Br J Obstet Gynaecol* 1987; **94:** 1192-1198.

145. Hirvonen E. Oral contraceptive containing oestradiol valerate for pre-menopausal women. In: Zichella L, Whitehead M, Van Keep PA, eds. *The Climacteric and Beyond.* Carnforth: Parthena Publishing Group, 1988; 118-121.

146. Watson NR, Studd JWW, Riddle AI, Savvas M. Suppression of ovulation by transdermal oestradiol patches. *Br Med J* 1988; **297:** 900-901.

11

INDEX

NOTE:
Since the major subject of this publication is "Hormone Replacement Therapy", limited references are to be found under this keyword, and readers are advised to seek more specific index entries.

12

12

12

12